The Epidural Epidemic

A Sensible Approach to Choosing Safe Pain Relief In Child Birth

Matthew Kumar, MD, JD

The Epidural Epidemic: A Sensible Approach to Choosing Safe Pain Relief In Childbirth
Published by Brikette House Publishing
Sunfish Lake, MN

ISBN: 979-8-9926716-0-5 (paperback)
ISBN: 979-8-9926716-1-2 (ebook)

HEALTH & FITNESS / Pregnancy & Childbirth

Interior and cover edited and designed by Danielle Anderson and the team at Ink Worthy Books. Publishing management by KLR Literary Management. Copyrights owned by Matthew Kumar, MD, JD.

Disclaimer: This book is not intended as a substitute for the medical advice of physicians. The reader should regularly consult a physician in matters relating to her health and particularly with respect to any symptoms that may require diagnosis or medical attention.

Quantity Purchases: Schools, companies, professional groups, clubs, and other organizations may qualify for special terms when ordering quantities of this title. For information, email the author at mmk47340@protonmail.com.

Contents

INTRODUCTION

It was a tense moment. The grandmother, her lips set in a hard line, made her stance clear. Through a Spanish translator, the nurse had tried every argument to persuade her:

"She'll be much more comfortable."

"This is just how we do it—everyone has an epidural."

"Look, the doctor is here, and he's waiting. We would rather not call him back when she changes her mind in the middle of the night."

But she was having none of it.

The young woman in labor, only 18 years old, is anxious and in pain, comprehending little of what is being said. Her mother is uncertain but clearly starting to cave under the pressure.

"We don't want it! Go away!" the grandmother tells the translator.

The nurse laughs derisively. "She doesn't want it? Okay, but she won't be able to handle the pain, and then when she asks for an epidural later, the doctor will be gone."

The girl and her mother quickly confer. "Okay!" gasps the girl. "Do it!"

Half an hour later, I drive home through the snow, knowing that, in all probability, I'll be called back in a matter of hours to do a cesarean section when the girl's labor stalls due to the epidural, endangering the baby—an unlikely event for a healthy 18-year-old giving birth without an epidural. I have seen such scenarios happen over and over again in my 40 years of practicing anesthesiology. I think about my sister, who runs a busy women's clinic in a large city in southern India. Her cesarean section rate is a tiny fraction of ours at this rural American hospital, yet her outcomes for mothers and babies are similar. I had never understood my sister's opposition to epidurals, but now I was beginning to wonder if she might be right.

At dawn, my pager goes off. "Failure of labor to progress." I return to the hospital to administer the anesthesia for the girl's C-section. I see the grandmother in the hallway, visibly worried; I avoid making eye contact with her.

Due to the nurse's persuasive abilities, the patient's insurance was billed twice for my services: once for the epidural and a second time for the C-section. The hospital profited as well. In fact, the entire medical system benefits from an increase in the cesarean section rate. Meanwhile, had the patient opted not to get an epidural, I would have never been involved in her care, and now a young mother and her baby face risks and long-term consequences that neither she nor her family had been prepared to consider.

Sadly, this situation is not fiction—it's a reality that's only increasing.

This scene, and countless others like it, have played out increasingly throughout my four decades in anesthesiology. Between 1965 and 1985, the cesarean section rate in the United States increased from 4.5 percent to 22.7 percent [1]. Today, the rate hovers around 32 percent [2]. This exponential rise in cesarean sections parallels the exponential rise in the use of epidurals. Once used sparingly, the use of epidurals rose from 22 percent in 1981 to nearly 80 percent by 2020 [3, 4].

Other than providing pain relief, the epidural offers little advantage to the mother or child. In contrast, we have seen a slew of skyrocketing adverse effects for mother and child, risks that are often understated, both immediate and delayed, emanating from epidurals.

Additionally, the cost of healthcare has concurrently exploded in proportion to the number of interventions, such as the epidural, on the mother and newborn. In 1978, a vaginal birth in New York City, with three days of hospital stay, was $1,500 [5]; but, in 2022, the average cost of a vaginal birth was $18,865, and the average cost of a cesarean birth was $26,280 [6].

Childbirth, though, is one of the most profound, natural processes in human life. Interestingly, childbirth is the only *nor-*

mal human physiological process that is associated with significant pain. Unlike a toothache, appendicitis, or kidney stone, there is no infection, inflammation, or obstruction causing the pain in childbirth. The process of labor is painful, even in the absence of disease, injury, or some other complication. Pain appears to be a necessary ingredient for healthy, normal childbirth, which triggers the release of oxytocin, a neuroendocrine hormone responsible for creating an unwavering bond between the mother and child. Hundreds of other physiological changes occur during pregnancy and labor that promote a healthy foundational start for the baby and prepare the mother for parenthood.

However, pain beyond one's limits of toleration can result in an unpleasant, emotionally draining experience for the woman and her family. To address this, modern medicine offers a wide array of pain relief options for women to choose from. Of these, the epidural is the most frequently chosen option, and astonishingly, it is often presented as though it's entirely risk-free, perfectly safe, and devoid of significant side effects. What actually happens, though, is that the obstetrician assumes that, prior to administering any pain medication, the anesthesiologist will discuss with the patient the available pain relief options and related risks. In contrast, on the day of labor, the anesthesiologist assumes the patient has already had discussions with her obstetrician so that she is able to make an informed decision. He would then only need to mention a few immediate complications to the patient before proceeding with the epidural. After all, the patient is in significant pain and needs immediate attention and not a discourse on the pros and cons of an epidural.

A discussion regarding the risks, benefits, and alternatives to the epidural should be held in the days and months before the due date, but sadly, it rarely is. Without this awareness, many women experience childbirth and receive epidurals without full knowledge of their potential to set off a cascade of complications, from prolonged labor to forceps delivery, perineal tears, and even issues affecting the baby's development.

This book aims to empower expectant mothers to make informed decisions about pain relief options during childbirth. It does not tell you what to choose but provides clear, evidence-based information about your options. The initial chapters explore the various methods of labor pain management, including their risks, complications, and long-term adverse effects on the mother and the child. Later in the book, I outline a four-step process to help you choose a childbirth labor pain approach tailored to your health, values, and unique circumstances.

This book will provide you with sufficient knowledge to confidently make your decision, well before your hospital visit. In addition to the four-step plan, the appendix includes a template for a birth plan. Use the document as a checklist to deliberate with your partner and healthcare provider to address the main issues you will encounter on the delivery day.

Thousands of women who have applied the four-step process I describe have gone on to experience soul-satisfying birthing and deliver healthy babies. They experience a sense of satisfaction in achieving a life's milestone with proper planning, control, and successful execution. Coming into the hospital with no birthing plan and not knowing what you want for yourself and the baby leaves your healthcare entirely to the mercy of your nurses and physicians, people who do their best to guide you but don't know your heart's desire.

On the day of delivery, no one will be sitting down with you to go over your pain relief options. Once the labor starts, you will do just about anything to mitigate the pain, and any intellectual discussion would be futile since your body and mind will be in survival mode. Therefore, you should decide in the comfort of your home, days, weeks, or even months before the anticipated delivery date.

An important objective of this book is to point out the real risks of labor pain options, and specifically the epidural. As you read through the options, you may discover that the epidural is the right choice for you. In fact, most women may decide on an epidural for labor pain management. And that would be appropriate for the vast majority. However, in a subset of women, the risks to the mother and baby from an epidural may far outweigh its benefits.

In the course of my medical practice and research, I have learned of several short- and long-term adverse effects of epidurals. The short-term adverse impacts are well known. However, the adverse long-term consequences are hidden in the medical literature. It's increasingly recognized that unnecessary interventions lead to unintended consequences. These adverse consequences are treated with further interventions, which lead to more complications. The idea that one intervention can lead to many more downstream ones is now known as a "cascade of interventions" [7, 8]. And indeed, the epidural kickstarts a cascade of interventions, as well as their unintended complications.

The complications of epidurals are like those of the Russian Matryoshka dolls (Figure 0-1). It looks like one simple complication, but 10 more are nestled within it. The epidural is like this—for example, it may prolong the labor, which can lead to a forceps delivery, which can cause a perineal tear, which can lead to urinary incontinence. The complications continue: the use of forceps can also cause trauma to the fetal head, which can lead to cerebral palsy, intracranial bleeding, or facial bone fracture. And there's more: the epidural is often chased with artificial augmentation of the labor with an oxytocin infusion, making the oxytocin administration itself another Matryoshka doll.

Many of the epidural's long-term adverse effects are unknown at this time. Some studies show impaired oxytocin levels in children with criminal antisocial behaviors, autism spectrum disorders (ASD), and impaired family bonding. There's considerable evidence that the use of epidurals, possibly combined with oxytocin infusion, is associated with a rise in children with ASD, in addition to attention-deficit/hyperactivity disorder (ADHD), anxiety, obsessive-compulsive disorder, and impaired speech, motor, and cognitive functions. Most of these adverse effects might not be recognized for several years until the child goes to school.

This book is designed to provide education on the various modalities of labor analgesia and help you make an informed decision. But the simple truth remains that humans have thrived for millennia without pain management during labor, specifically the epidural. Even today, most of the world's population gives birth without access to labor analgesia and achieves healthy outcomes. My goal with this book is not to vilify the epidural but to advocate for balanced, informed decision-making. By understanding the whole picture, you can make the best choice for yourself and your baby—one that aligns with your values, protects your health, and ensures a positive, empowering birthing experience.

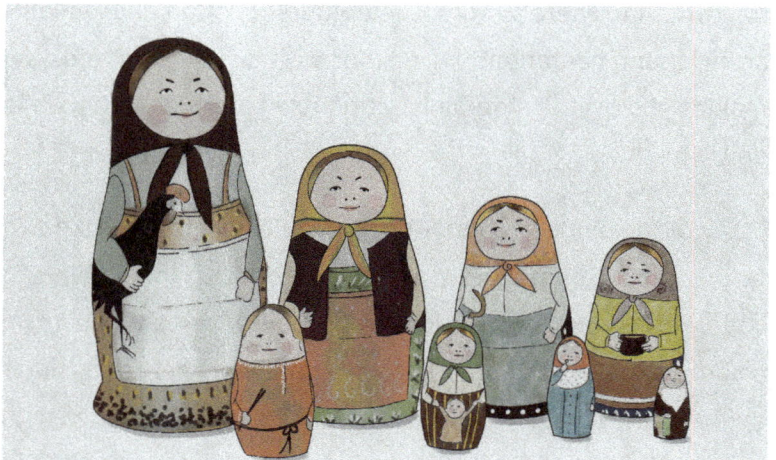

Figure 0-1. Russian Matryoshka dolls. Like these dolls, many other complications are often nestled within epidural complications.

Chapter 1

THE NATURE OF LABOR PAIN

You are here because you want to learn more about pain management options to make an informed decision when you are in labor. Research shows that women empowered with knowledge and support are more likely to navigate the complexities of childbirth with confidence and clarity, leading to healthier maternal and neonatal experiences [9, 10]. Comprehensive childbirth education alleviates anxiety and leads to better health outcomes during pregnancy and delivery [10]. With increased access to information and support systems, women can develop self-care skills that enhance their overall well-being and contribute positively to reproductive health outcomes [11].

Neuroanatomy of Labor Pain

Let's start with a clear understanding of the neuroanatomy of labor pain, which will aid in your grasp of how modern interventions and medications work to block the pain pathways. Much like electricity traveling along wires, pain sensations travel in peripheral nerves in waves of cell depolarization from the limbs, body, and organs to nerve cell clusters in the spinal cord and then to the brain. Their spread can be blocked anywhere along this pathway with medications such as local anesthetics.

Labor pain is perceived in the brain as intense, spasmodic, stretching, and agonizing—and rightly so. Most women will describe their first labor as the worst pain of their lives. Yet each woman's labor is unique, and each woman experiences pain somewhat differently. Thankfully for many women, the pain does tend to diminish in intensity with each subsequent birth. After the fifth child, spinal interventions as a solution for pain management are rarely necessary.

For humans, pregnancy lasts on average 280 days (40 weeks), calculated from the onset of a woman's last menstrual period. Nearly 80 percent of women will deliver within 10 days of this estimated delivery date. Once the baby is sufficiently grown and matured within the uterus, stretch signals from the uterus and hormonal changes in the mother precipitate labor. To expel the baby from the uterus into the outside world, the uterus must contract vigorously, and the birth canal needs to stretch and dilate to allow the baby's passage during birth.

This physiological process leads to two distinct types of pain during labor: (1) colicky pain, which is abdominal pain that tends to come and go in waves and is caused by the muscular contraction of the uterus (what are referred to as "contractions") and (2) stretching pain from the fetus stretching the birth canal.

The colicky pain from contractions starts as mild in intensity and duration, spaced five to seven minutes apart, then gradually grows more intense, lasting almost a minute and coming two to three minutes apart. The stretching pain is caused by the dilatation of the cervix, vagina, vulva, pelvic floor muscles, and the ligaments of the pelvic joints, and it is constant, aching, and persists until the delivery of the fetus.

Figure 1-1 illustrates the source of pain during labor and how various analgesic interventions block pain perception, which we'll cover in the following chapters.

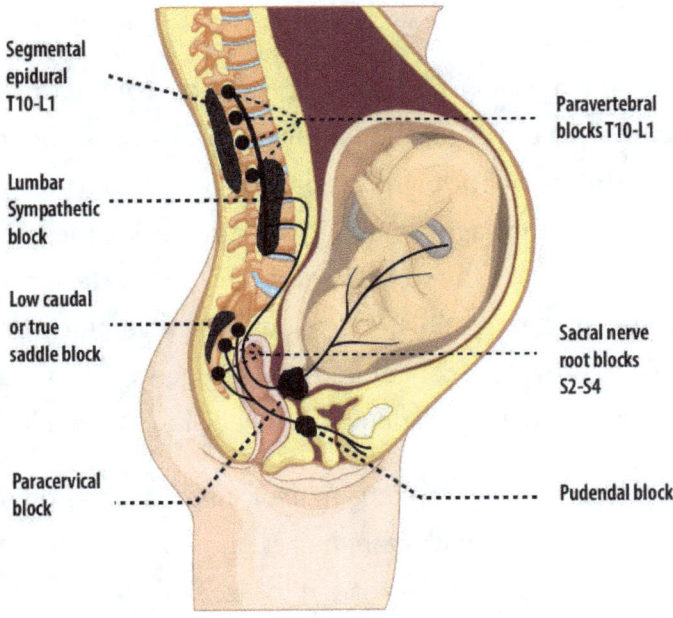

Figure 1-1. Diagram of the innervations of the uterus and the birth canal. The sites of various nerve blocks are shown.

The colicky pain from the contraction of the uterus is sometimes referred to as visceral pain. Sympathetic nervous system fibers carry the pain impulses to the spinal cord at the levels of T10-T11-T12-L1. This is the reason an epidural or spinal block performed at these levels in the spine is quite effective in interrupting a laboring mother's pain perceptions. Your obstetrician or the anesthesiologist could also inject local anesthetic through the fornix of the vagina, just lateral to the cervix, at the three and nine o'clock positions, to anesthetize the sensory fibers of the uterus, cervix, and upper vagina before they reach the spine. This injection is called a "paracervical block" and can be effective in controlling visceral pain.

The stretching pain that results from the descent of the fetal head through the vagina and perineal muscles is sometimes referred to as somatic pain. The pain impulses from the lower two-thirds of the vagina and perineum travel via the pudendal nerves to reach the spinal cord at the S2-S3-S4 levels. Your obstetrician can administer a pudendal nerve block transvaginal to provide excellent perineal analgesia. This block is effective for low-forceps delivery and episiotomy repair.

Intravenously administered pain medications such as opioids, dexmedetomidine, and ketamine act primarily at the level of the brain and, to a small extent, at the level of the spinal cord. The bloodstream carries them and reaches the pain-relaying nuclei in the brain's thalamus, blocking the transmission of pain impulses to the cortical centers to perceive pain. They have also been shown to affect pain transmission at the level of the posterior horn of the grey matter of the spinal cord, thereby mitigating the intensity of pain sensations that reach the brain.

Generally speaking, while we can't stop labor from being painful, Figure 1-1 shows that options do exist to minimize or eliminate the feeling of that pain. The most effective means to block the pain sensations from reaching your brain is by blocking the conduction of sensations at the level of the spine, either through an epidural or spinal injection of local anesthetics. In the subsequent chapters, we will review how an epidural or spinal analgesia is performed.

Pain Versus Suffering During Childbirth

It is important to understand that pain and suffering are separate and distinct experiences. This might seem unusual, so let's explore the concept further. Suffering is closely related to how we perceive and experience life. Depending on the intensity and nature of suffering, we may feel varying levels of satisfaction or dissatisfaction, as well as happiness or sorrow. For instance, it is common for someone to exercise intensely and experience physical pain, yet still find satisfaction in the process, often due to the benefits of improved physical health. This can be viewed as the secondary gain from pain. Achieving one's goals may also involve some suffering, but it can ultimately lead to happiness.

When we experience pain, it is processed and interpreted in a few specific areas of the brain. Figure 1-2 maps out the flow of pain through the processing centers in the brain. As you can see, neuroscience indicates that the sensation of pain from physical strain is processed in the thalamus of the brain. The limbic system then further interprets this pain as aversion, dissatisfaction, satisfaction, or acceptance. Finally, the prefrontal cortex processes this information from the limbic system into feelings of happiness or sorrow.

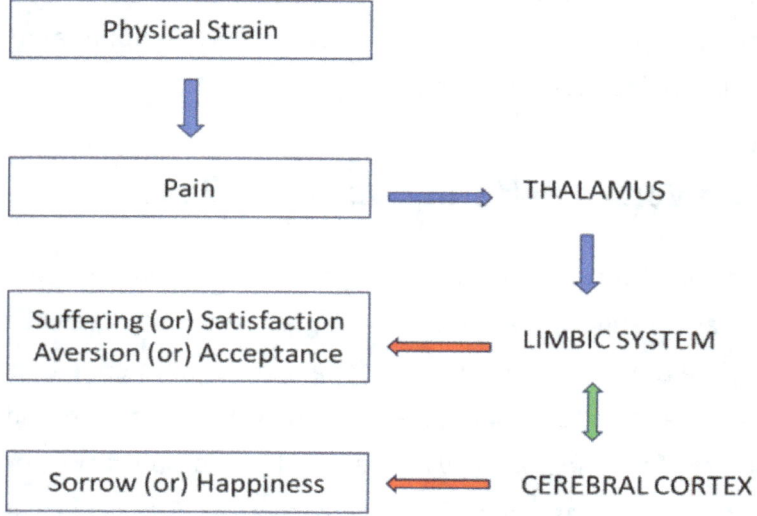

Figure 1-2. The perception of pain occurs at the level of the thalamus, while its characterization as sorrow or happiness occurs at the level of the cerebral cortex.

Hence, it's not at all uncommon for mothers who have experienced significant pain during natural childbirth to express immense satisfaction and feel happy after a birth. On the other hand, women who receive excellent pain relief from epidurals sometimes express suffering and dissatisfaction following the birthing process. They express sorrow and depression despite experiencing little or no pain during labor. Simply stated, your ability to have a satisfactory childbirth experience is not necessarily directly related to the level of pain you experience.

In fact, scientific studies validate the lack of correlation between maternal satisfaction and the magnitude of pain relief [12]. The key factors influencing how birthing pain is experienced include one's expectations, religious beliefs, moral and ethical values, childhood experiences, cultural norms, and the presence or absence of supportive family members. Recently, a young Yazidi mother gave birth in a hospital but refused all medical interventions, including an IV. Throughout her labor, her family and extended family visited her frequently, providing loving moral support. Despite experiencing significant pain, the birthing experience was a joyous occasion for her. To celebrate, the girl's father purchased expensive Turkish sweets for the entire birthing unit at the hospital.

Therefore, it is essential to understand that experiencing pain during childbirth does not mean you will have an unsatisfactory birthing experience. Rather, your best experience will likely result from embracing the pain and adjusting your expectations to acknowledge that discomfort is a part of labor. By doing this, you can go through the process with a sense of accomplishment and ultimately experience happiness.

Chapter 2

EPIDURAL ANALGESIA

The first pain relief option for expectant mothers that we will discuss is epidural analgesia, also known as the "epidural."

The invention of continuous lumbar epidural analgesia was one of the most important advancements in obstetrics in the 20th century. It has provided reliable pain relief and comfort during labor for more women than any other intervention. It has transformed childbirth from a much-feared, formidable, life-changing experience into an emotionally satisfying, tolerable, purposeful, controlled event. In the United States, nearly 80 percent of White, 70 percent of Black, and 65 percent of Hispanic women opted for epidural analgesia during childbirth from 2010 to 2017. These numbers continue to increase every year.

How the Epidural Is Performed

The epidural is performed by carefully placing a needle in the spine and advancing it until the potential space, called the epidural space, is reached (see Figure 2-1).

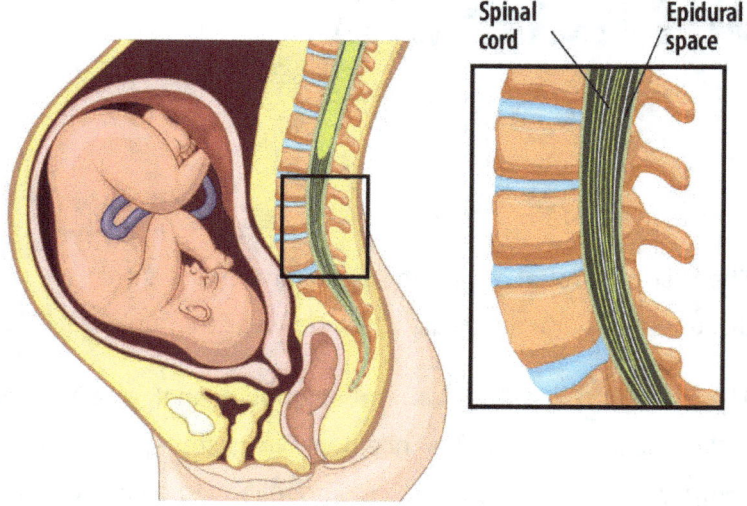

Figure 2-1. Anatomical location of the epidural space.

Then, a thin plastic catheter is inserted through the needle into the space, and the needle is removed. The catheter is secured to the back with adhesive tape, which is then used to infuse local anesthetic into the spine. The local anesthetic blocks the transmission of pain sensations emanating from the uterus and the birth canal from reaching the spinal cord. Because the neuronal pathways in the spinal cord connect to the brain, the patient perceives no pain.

The anesthesiologist can infuse a very dilute concentration of local anesthetic to block just the pain sensation nerve fibers. The medication commonly used in an epidural is bupivacaine 0.125 percent solution. The nerve fibers responsible for motor functions, such as muscle tone and the ability to move your limbs, are spared at this low concentration. Thus, while there will be minor motor weakness in your pelvic and lower limb muscles, you can still move your limbs while the pain is blocked.

If maintaining mobility is a primary concern, some anesthesiologists will use bupivacaine 0.0625 percent, a dilute concentration that tends to block only the pain-conducting nerve fibers and spare the motor nerves. This is often referred to as the "walking epidural" because the mother can still walk while enjoying pain relief. However, because the response to drugs is usually a bell-curve distribution, even at very low concentrations, the local anesthetics could cause significant motor weakness in some laboring mothers. Anesthesiologists often add tiny amounts of opioid medications to the local anesthetic infusion to improve the density of the sensory block without worsening motor weakness. The opioid medications are thought to diffuse through the membranes covering the spinal cord and block the pain sensations at the dorsal horn of the spinal cord.

In my own experience, however, seldom have I seen walking epidurals offer any real pain relief. In addition, walking epidurals always carry a risk of falls and significant harm to the mother and baby when they actually attempt to walk with an epidural in place. If pain relief is the primary objective, it is best to stick with a conventional epidural (which comes with medications such as bupivacaine 0.125 percent with fentanyl 1 ug/ml or ropiva-caine 0.2 percent with fentanyl 1 ug/ml). If you're having your first baby, unless you enjoy suffering all the complications of an epidural with little to marginal pain relief, you should stay away from walking epidurals. They sound great in theory, but while many publications are currently touting their virtues, they are rarely effective in clinical practice.

Advantages

The significant advantage of epidural analgesia is the pre-dictability of adequate analgesia. Unlike other modalities, such as intravenous pain medications, paracervical block, or inhala-tion of nitrous oxide, a well-placed epidural will guarantee ef-fective and immediate pain relief. Epidurals also allow the anesthesiologist to adjust the care based on your specific needs, including your body's build and shape, as well as your pain tolerance. This is done by adjusting the density and spinal level of the block as needed.

For example, to achieve better pain relief, the spinal level can be easily increased from L2 to T10 or even higher by merely increasing the local anesthetic bolus (volume of medication). In some patients, despite adequate spinal level, the quality or density of sensory block might not be adequate to achieve sat-isfactory pain relief. Under these circumstances, a small amount of highly concentrated local anesthetic (usually 3-5 ml of bupi-vacaine or ropivacaine 0.5 percent or even 1 percent) could be injected to increase the density of the block for breakthrough episodes of pain.

Because the level of spinal analgesia can be controlled and increased incrementally, precipitous blood pressure and heart rate drops are less frequent with epidurals than with intrathecal spinal injections. An epidural catheter placed with adequate antiseptic precautions can often be left in place for 48 to 72 hours without fear of infection.

Furthermore, should a cesarean section become necessary, epidural analgesia can easily accommodate this need. An epidural can be converted to epidural anesthesia by injecting a higher concentration of local anesthetic to increase the density of sensory block and induce motor blockade of the lower abdominal, pelvic, and lower limb muscles, which is necessary for a cesarean section procedure. Usually, 2 percent lidocaine with 1:200,000 epinephrine or 3 percent chloroprocaine is used to convert epidural analgesia into anesthesia.

For these reasons, continuous lumbar epidural analgesia is the most frequently used pain relief modality in the Western world.

Disadvantages

One of the more practical disadvantages of an epidural is that performing the procedure and establishing adequate pain relief takes time. Depending on the anatomy of the spine and the experience of the anesthesiologist, it could take anywhere from 20 to 90 minutes to achieve a satisfactory epidural block. In contrast, achieving a spinal block with an intrathecal injection (otherwise known as a "spinal," which we'll cover in detail in a future chapter) is much easier and much faster. Most providers can perform a spinal block in 10 to 20 minutes. Thus, if your labor is too far along, an epidural may not be an option for you.

Another disadvantage of the epidural is the potential for life-long adverse effects on the fetus. Despite denunciations from the medical establishment, credible studies are showing a strong correlation between epidurals and the occurrence of autism, ADHD, and lack of bonding in children born under epidural analgesia. We will look further into these adverse effects shortly.

And, of course, a significant disadvantage of epidurals is the complications to the mother, as listed in Table 2-1 below.

Epidural Maternal Complication	Occurrence Rate
Maternal hypotension	80/100
Maternal hypoventilation	20/100
Fetal heart rate abnormality	20/100
Maternal bradycardia	15/100
PDPH	1/100
Transient neurological injury	1/6,700
Spinal infection	1/145,000
Spinal hematoma	1/168,000
Persistent neurological injury	1/240,000
Cardiac arrest	1/40,000–1/460,000
Maternal death	2.5/1,000,000–3.8/1,000,000

Table 2-1. Maternal complications of epidural.

Often, complications are increased in women with spinal deformities, edema from eclampsia, obesity, and prior surgical interventions on the spine. Under these conditions, it's difficult for the anesthesiologist to properly place the epidural catheter and administer the local anesthetics in the correct location. Nerve injury can occur from the needle tip inadvertently piercing a spinal nerve root or from injection of local anesthetic into the nerve itself (intraneural injection). The insult to the nerve can be either temporary (referred to as "transient" in Table 2-1) or permanent (referred to as "persistent" in Table 2-1), resulting in sensory loss, pain, and weakness in the lower extremities and pelvis.

The needle can also puncture a blood vessel in the spine and lead to intraspinal bleeding, which could be slow and lead to a delay in recognition of an epidural, intrathecal, or intramedullary hematoma (a swelling of clotted blood within the tissues). If a spinal hematoma is not promptly recognized and the bleeding is not stopped, it can cause compression of the spinal cord and spinal nerves, leading to paralysis in the lower limbs and loss of bladder and bowel control.

Inserting a needle into the spine also risks seeding bacteria from the skin surface or the needle itself into deeper spine tissues. Spinal infection can occur beneath the skin or between the meningeal coverings of the spine or infect the cerebrospinal fluid. If not promptly recognized and treated, spinal infection can lead to nerve palsy, paralysis, or death. Spinal infections are frequent when the provider is forced to hurry and has insufficient time to prepare the skin or follow sterile procedures adequately. This is one good reason not to wait until you are later in stage one labor, with the cervix dilated eight centimeters or greater, when the contractions are intense and frequent, and you're screaming for immediate pain relief.

Other complications, such as nerve injury and a post-dural puncture headache ("PDPH"), are also more frequent when the epidural is hurried and performed later in the first stage of labor.

Proximate Adverse Effects

In addition to the complications discussed in the previous section, some adverse effects of the epidural are not immediately apparent, and the chain of events that follows can obscure the causal link between the epidural and these negative outcomes. Nevertheless, these adverse effects are genuine, caused by the epidural, and can result in long-term issues for both the mother and the child. The following discussion will outline some of the more common immediate adverse effects. These complications are unlikely to occur without the use of an epidural.

Prolongation of Labor

Epidurals cause a loss of sensation and muscle weakness in the lower abdomen and pelvis. This makes it difficult for the mother to strain and push the fetus out, as she cannot feel where and how she is pushing. Obstetricians often start an oxytocin infusion to counteract the delay in stage one labor when an epidural is used. In such cases, many studies show a prolongation of all stages of labor, but especially stage two. This delay often results in the application of forceps or a vacuum extractor to deliver the baby. Additionally, a large episiotomy, or surgical cut, is usually needed to facilitate the application of the forceps.

In the worst case, the obstetrician might decide to perform a cesarean section to deliver the baby. Prolonged labor can lead to serious infection and increase the risk of postpartum bleeding. Long-term adverse effects of prolongation of labor include pelvic floor muscle damage in the mother, leading later in life to urinary incontinence and prolapse of the rectum, bladder, or uterus. Prolonged labor also adversely affects the fetus. Studies show there can be a rise in fetal infection rates, fetal distress, and perinatal hypoxemia, all of which can cause neurological injury to the brain with long-term adverse consequences.

Increased Probability of Cesarean Section

While there are conflicting studies on whether epidurals increase the probability of C-section deliveries, I firmly believe they do. Common sense will lead you to the correct conclusion—when the woman cannot push due to muscle weakness caused by the epidural, there are only two options: either to apply forceps and pull the fetus out or perform a C-section and deliver the baby through the abdomen. Unfortunately, authors of studies that do find an increased incidence of C-sections in epidural patients are often reluctant to state the truth and try to rationalize the findings with other improbable factors [13].

Increased Probability of Forceps Delivery

Weakness and numbness caused by the epidural impair fetal descent and the mother's ability to push. As a result, obstetricians are often forced to resort to forceps or vacuum extractors to deliver babies. Again, some studies show no difference in forceps usage between women who had an epidural and those who didn't. In my experience, there has been a significant increase in the use of forceps in expectant mothers with epidurals.

The application of forceps is not without complications. Forceps can cause trauma to fetal facial bones, eyes, ears, nose, and dental ridges. More seriously, they can cause skull fractures, contusions, or lacerations of the brain. Severe brain injury can occur from bleeding and hematoma formation inside the skull. In extreme cases, fetal death can occur from excessive traction on the neck and brainstem. The case study in the following section (Figure 2-2) is an extreme example of decapitation from excessive pulling on the fetal head.

Increased Probability of Episiotomy

Weakness and numbness caused by the epidural also impair the fetal head rotation and descent. This often requires an episiotomy, with or without forceps, to deliver the baby. Many studies confirm the increased use of episiotomy in patients treated with epidural analgesia [14-16]. Again, this increased incidence of episiotomy makes sense when one realizes that the epidural makes the lower abdominal and pelvic muscles weak, so much so that the fetal head has to be pulled or pushed out by the obstetrician. An episiotomy enlarges the vaginal outlet making it easier to push the head out, either by applying pressure over the lower abdomen or applying forceps or a vacuum extractor to pull the head out.

Increased Use of Oxytocin Infusion

Most often, oxytocin infusion is started to correct "dynamic dystocia" or failure of labor progression due to poor uterine contraction and stagnant cervical dilatation. This happens because the epidural blocks the uterine nerve signals reaching the brain. The brain, devoid of stimulation, turns down the release of intrinsic oxytocin, relaxin, and other neural hormones necessary for the natural progression of labor. Essentially, the brain does not register that the woman is in labor, so it does not release the essential hormones to help it along, thus requiring the doctor to provide the oxytocin infusion needed.

In addition, the relaxation of pelvic and lower abdominal muscles thwarts the mother's ability to push with each contraction.

Unfortunately, the artificial contractions produced by the oxytocin infusion could result in uterine rupture, particularly if the mother had a prior C-section. Once on oxytocin infusion, it is also a customary practice to rupture the membranes. The membranes act as a barrier to the invasion of microbes. Without their integrity, infection of the uterus and the fetus will likely occur if the delivery is not completed within six to 12 hours.

Oxytocin infusion is not recommended in situations involving fetal malposition, cephalo-pelvic disproportion, and placenta previa. The risks to the fetus from massive doses of oxytocin entering its circulation are only now being studied. Lack of mother-child bonding, antisocial behaviors, and ASD are thought to be some of the long-term adverse effects on the child.

Immediate Adverse Effects On the Fetus

A serious immediate risk of epidural is the propensity to cause fetal distress, a condition where the fetal brain is starved of oxygen. The epidural can precipitate fetal distress by either causing low blood pressure in the mother or causing anesthetic medications to enter the fetal circulation. Both insults to the fetus can cause death or significant brain injury if not promptly corrected.

The uterus receives approximately 500 to 700 ml per minute of blood flow during labor. When the epidural causes low blood pressure, the perfusion of the placenta can drop as a result, depriving the fetus of the much-needed oxygen and nutrients. A distressed fetus can compensate for a lack of oxygen for a few minutes. However, if the reduction is significant (under 50 percent) and lasts several minutes, it can lead to hypoxia and acidosis in the fetus. The lack of oxygen is reflected in fetal heart rate abnormalities and acidosis in fetal scalp blood samples (pH under 7.20).

Under these circumstances, the obstetrician should take measures to correct the cause of hypoxia or proceed to deliver the baby operatively. In many cases, the nonreassuring fetal heart rhythms are corrected by simple measures such as administration of oxygen to the mother, repositioning the mother to alleviate aortocaval compression, or administering IV fluids or inotropic medications.

The anesthetic medications used in the epidural can cross the placental circulation and enter the fetal circulation with immediate adverse effects. Local anesthetic agents such as bupivacaine have been shown to cause significant constriction of the umbilical artery. In a fetus that is already compromised due to maternal hypotension, further reduction in umbilical artery blood flow can worsen hypoxia and acidosis.

Opioid medications administered to the mother through the epidural can accumulate in sufficient quantities in the fetus. They pose little threat to the fetus as long as the fetus remains in the uterus and the placental circulation is active. However, upon birth, they will render the baby weak, sedated, poorly responsive, and slow to begin spontaneous respiration. The obstetrician must immediately counteract the effects of the opioids with naloxone or be ready to insert an endotracheal tube and provide mechanical ventilation for the newborn. Any delay in resuscitation of a sedated baby could lead to profound hypoxic brain injury.

Long-Term Adverse Effects On the Newborn

By increasing the risk of operative and forceps deliveries, epidurals predispose the babies to trauma from instruments and toxicity from anesthetic agents. However, more recent studies point to the development of autism and other neuropsychiatric developmental disorders in the offspring of women birthing under epidural.

The medical literature remains unsettled. The causal connections are difficult to study due to the ethical and logistical issues in creating near-identical prospective treatment and control groups. Nevertheless, some studies are shedding light on this issue. We will examine them in the next chapter.

Case Study: An Unintended Consequence of Epidural and Forceps

The following case study is an extreme example of decapitation from excessive pulling on the fetal head. Unfortunately, epidurals numb the perineum, and the laboring mother will not feel the pain and be able to provide feedback to the obstetrician when excessive force is applied through the use of forceps, causing significant damage to the mother and baby.

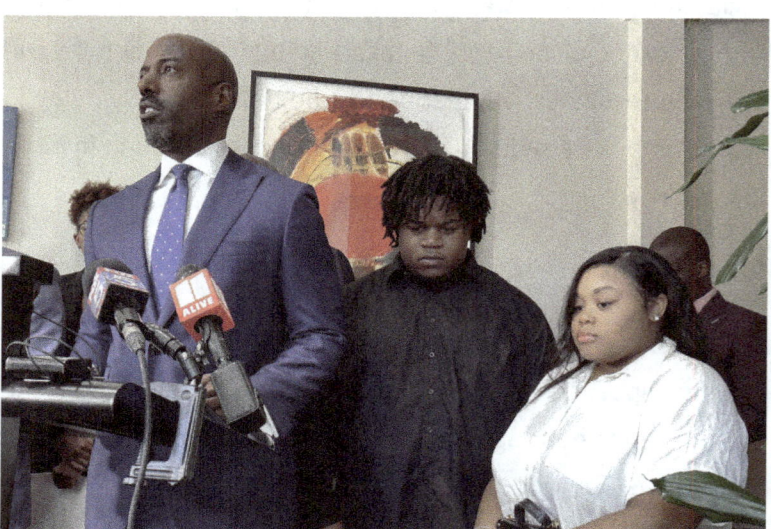

Figure 2-2. Ms. Jessica Ross, who lost her baby due to excessive traction from forceps, and her partner, at a news conference with their attorney. (Copyright 2023, Sudhin Thanawala / AP).

The lawsuit of *Jessica Ross v. Tracey St. Julian, MD,* involves allegations against obstetrician Tracey St. Julian and Southern Regional Medical Center in Atlanta, Georgia, regarding a tragic childbirth incident on July 9, 2023. Jessica Ross was admitted for labor and delivery and given oxytocin, but complications arose due to shoulder dystocia, preventing the baby from descending correctly during delivery. The obstetrician attempted several techniques, including forceps, vacuum extraction, manual traction, and an episiotomy.

At 10:36 p.m., the fetal heart rate showed critical distress, and by 10:46 p.m., the baby had no detectable heartbeat. The lawsuit claims that excessive traction applied by the obstetrician resulted in the baby's decapitation. A subsequent cesarean section delivered the torso and legs at 12:11 a.m., followed by the decapitated head vaginally. An autopsy revealed severe trauma, including skull fractures, brain injuries, cervical spine damage, and spinal cord rupture.

The lawsuit also alleges attempts to conceal the decapitation, with the hospital reportedly discouraging an autopsy, suggesting cremation, and presenting the baby to the parents in a manner designed to hide the injuries.

The hospital denied all allegations, citing privacy laws, but expressed condolences while reaffirming its commitment to quality care. Attorney Cory Lynch emphasized the devastating impact on the grieving parents, who had anticipated the birth of their first child.

Chapter 3

THE EPIDURAL AND THE RISK OF AUTISM

The possible complications that could impact your unborn child are a crucial factor to consider when deciding whether to choose an epidural. While we have touched upon some potential complications to the fetus in the preceding chapter, it is important to delve deeper into this issue.

Specifically, this chapter will take a look at certain neuropsychiatric disorders. Although not yet settled science, several well-conducted studies demonstrate a significant correlation between the use of epidurals and the incidence of autism spectrum disorder (ASD) in children [17-24].

Not only is there a correlation between the epidural and ASD, but there's also an association with specific developmental disorders, ADHD, intellectual disability, and epilepsy in offspring. The association, though, is most substantial for autism.

The available evidence for a correlation between epidural and autism can be grouped under three separate categories:

1. Global occurrence of autism and the rates of epidural

2. Retrospective studies of offspring of women with and without epidural

3. Retrospective studies of offspring of women who received oxytocin

However, before proceeding, you must understand that correlation does not necessarily imply causation. For example, there's a strong correlation between high blood pressure and a stroke. Does high blood pressure cause a stroke? Or is it the stiffening of arteries by atherosclerosis that causes both high blood pressure and a stroke? The answer depends on the nature of the variables and the strength of interactions between them. Correlation may portend a causal relationship, but it's not always necessarily true. Be sure to keep that in mind as we continue our discussion.

Another critical factor to consider is the motive of the medical-pharmaceutical industrial complex. Your obstetrician, nurse, anesthesiologist, hospital, and pharmaceutical company all stand to gain financially from you having an epidural. A quietly resting patient means less work for the nurse and the obstetrician. The longer the epidural lasts, the more money the anesthesiologist and the pharmacist get to bill for their services and products, and the patient is happy with her pain-free labor. This arrangement appears to be a win-win situation for all parties involved. However, this collaboration neglects to include the silent victim: the baby. The baby might not know until much later in their life that their mother's labor analgesia choice was the root cause of their disability. And it is they who must live with a crippling neuropsychiatric disorder for the remainder of their life.

As we look at the data behind the potential correlation between epidural and autism rates, there are a few things to keep in mind. Studies that attempt to disprove the correlation between epidural and autism or other neuropsychiatric disorders must be taken with a grain of salt. There's too much secondary gain for physicians, nurses, hospitals, and pharmaceutical companies to give up epidurals completely. Even studies that intend to disprove correlation often find their raw data showing the existence of correlation. Then, only through spurious statistical analysis and the introduction of additional variables (confounding variables) can they claim the correlation is insignificant. Let's take a closer look.

Global Occurrence of Autism and the Rates of Epidural

When one looks at the rates of autism in the US, we see they are highest in the Northeast, the West Coast, and Minnesota. These are also the states with the highest utilization rates for epidurals. It is also clear that in states with increasing usage of epidurals, there is a concurrent rise in the rate of autism. Since 2019, due to the widespread migration of undocumented aliens, the statistics have been somewhat distorted. Still, in every state, the rise in epidural utilization is associated with an increase in autism.

In examining World Health Organization data, it is evident that technologically advanced nations, located mostly in North America and Europe, have the highest rates of epidurals. Lesser advanced developing countries in Asia and Africa show significantly lower rates of epidurals.

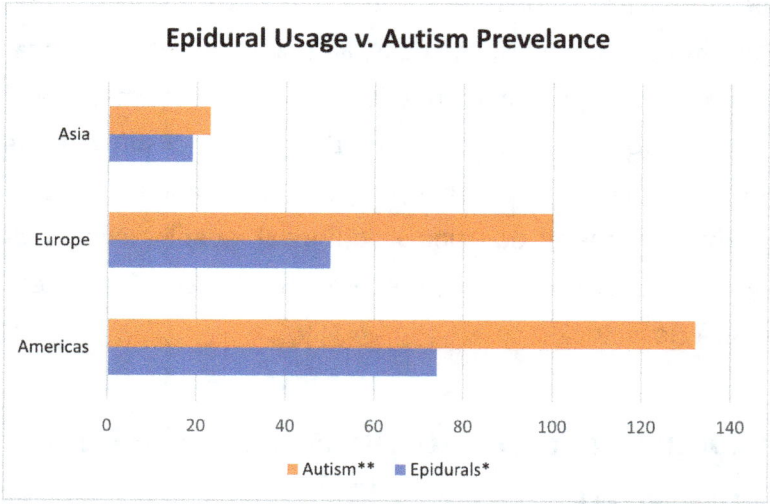

Figure 3-1. Data synthesized from World Health Organization publications. Comparing ASD per 10,000 children and epidural per 100 parturients.

When autism rates from different countries are collated and superimposed on available data on epidural usage, there is a striking correlation between the use of epidurals and the occurrence of autism (see Figure 3-1). In China, where the epidural rates are rising, the occurrence of autism is also increasing.

Retrospective Studies of Offspring of Women With and Without Epidural

Some excellent studies look backward in time to examine the relationship between an intervention or exposure to a drug and the outcomes in two or more distinct groups. Let us examine one study that showed a 37 percent increased risk of autism with epidurals [23]. The study looked at nearly 148,000 children born by vaginal delivery at 28 to 44 weeks gestation in Kaiser Permanente Southern California hospitals between 2008 and 2015. Autism spectrum disorders were diagnosed in 2,039 children (1.9 percent) in the epidural group and 485 children (1.3 percent) in the non-epidural group.

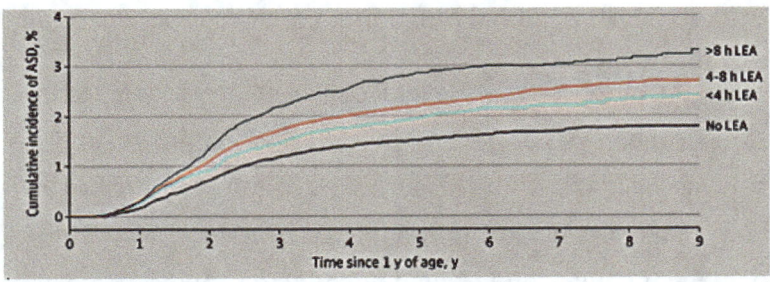

Figure 3-2. Relationship between epidural and the occurrence of autism. Increasing levels of exposure leads to increasing levels of adverse outcomes.

This study, as one can see from Figure 3-2, not only showed a strong correlation between epidurals and autism, but it also showed a dose-response effect. This means the longer the mother was treated with an epidural (under four hours versus four to eight hours versus over eight hours), the more likely the incidence of autism. Now, that is convincing evidence of a causal relationship between the two variables: epidurals and autism. In addition, the graph suggests the autism curves were continuing to curve upward at age nine when the study was concluded, implying that, if the children had been followed for a more extended period, more cases of autism would have been discovered.

Now let's look at a study that is supposed to have put this controversy to rest and declared no correlation between epidurals and autism [19]. This study is said to have looked at the incidence of autism in 479,178 Danish children born with or without epidurals. Unfortunately, contrary to their expectations, the raw data from the study showed a significant difference in autism between children born with epidurals and those born naturally.

Then, the authors added several confounding variables to their statistical analysis and found the correlation minimal and statistically insignificant (see Figure 3-3). They added 20 or so variables, such as smoking, obesity, education, geography, and so on, which could potentially have affected the occurrence of autism. It's commonly known in the field of statistics that data can be manipulated to achieve the desired outcome by adding variables that make a correlation appear or disappear. I am not here to tell you what to believe. Instead, I will let you decide on the accuracy of this study's conclusion by analyzing both its crude and adjusted data.

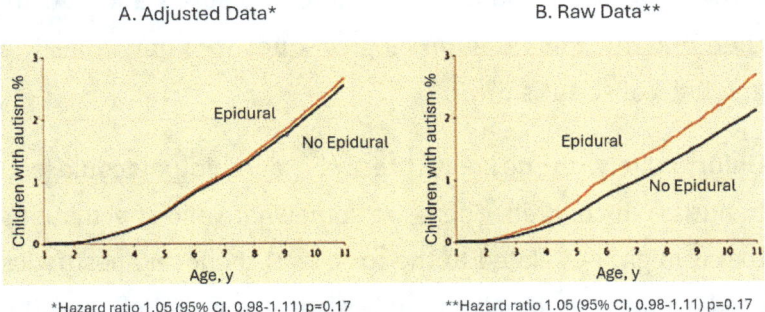

*Hazard ratio 1.05 (95% CI, 0.98-1.11) p=0.17   **Hazard ratio 1.05 (95% CI, 0.98-1.11) p=0.17

Figure 3-3. Data showing differences in the occurrence of autism between epidural and non-epidural groups. A) Adjusted for confounding variables. B) Raw data.

Looking at the data, I'm not convinced the correlation between epidurals and autism disappears when confounding variables are added. It's difficult to see why the investigators would have added the confounding variables other than to adjust the data results, because the raw data did not support what they set out to prove. While you should draw your own conclusions, in my opinion, the most crucial element of this study is the raw data, which shows a clear and convincing correlation between the use of epidurals and the occurrence of autism. Adding confounding variables, such as smoking, race, education, socioeconomic status, height, weight, age, and similar variables, can annul almost any correlation in most studies, making it act as a secret weapon used to sabotage a conclusion one does not like—it becomes a means to deal with an inconvenient truth.

How Does an Epidural Cause Autism?

If there's a causal connection between epidurals and autism, then one must ask the next logical question: how does the epidural cause autism?

Unfortunately, no one knows precisely how epidurals could lead to autism in children. There are somewhat valid speculations that it might be related to the toxicity of the local anesthetics used in epidurals. Small amounts of local anesthetics enter the fetus through the placenta and reach the fetal brain. It's hypothesized that the immature developing brain is more susceptible to the toxic effects of local anesthetics than adult brains. These changes in the developing brain may include abnormalities in synaptogenesis, neurogenesis, and neuronal apoptosis. These neurotoxic effects have been observed at concentrations used in clinical practice and are known to alter normal behavioral development in newborn rhesus monkeys [25].

However, while this theory has some merit, the neurotoxicity of the local anesthetics might not be the sole culprit. It's more likely the result of a lack of sufficient oxygen supply to the fetal brain. Brain cells, particularly developing ones, are highly susceptible to even a brief lack of oxygen (hypoxia).

To appreciate how delicately the brain depends on oxygen supply, let us review what we already know about the effects of hypoxia on the brain. In the adult, loss of consciousness ensues after 60 to 90 seconds of lack of oxygen, permanent unconsciousness sets in after two to three minutes, the brain loses all electrical activity after three to four minutes, and irreversible programmed cell death ensues after five to seven minutes. This hypoxia-induced cell death preferentially affects the brain's most oxygen-dependent regions, such as the cerebral cortex, hippocampus, basal ganglion, and cerebellum. Thus, while the brain survives under hypoxic conditions, it manifests residual neurological deficits. Oxygen deprivation brings about a spectrum of neurological injuries, ranging from very mild functional deficits to cell death in different regions of the hypoxic brain. This is probably what happens to the fetus under epidural anesthesia.

The next logical question, then, is **how the epidural causes fetal hypoxia.** Let's explore this next.

When a woman receives an epidural, the local anesthetics she is given not only block the sensory signals from the pelvis and lower limbs, thus blocking the pain, but they also block the efferent sympathetic nerves that maintain muscle tone in the blood vessels and stimulate the heart to contract. The sympathetic nerves are closely integrated with the spinal nerves in the thoracic and lumbar sections of the spinal cord (see Figure 3-4). This chemically induced "sympathectomy" causes vasodilation in the lower half of the body and slows the heart rate and contractility. The resulting lack of sympathetic stimulation causes an abnormal heart rhythm (bradycardia) and low blood pressure (hypotension), with blood pooling in the lower limbs and pelvis. This causes the cardiac output to decline as well.

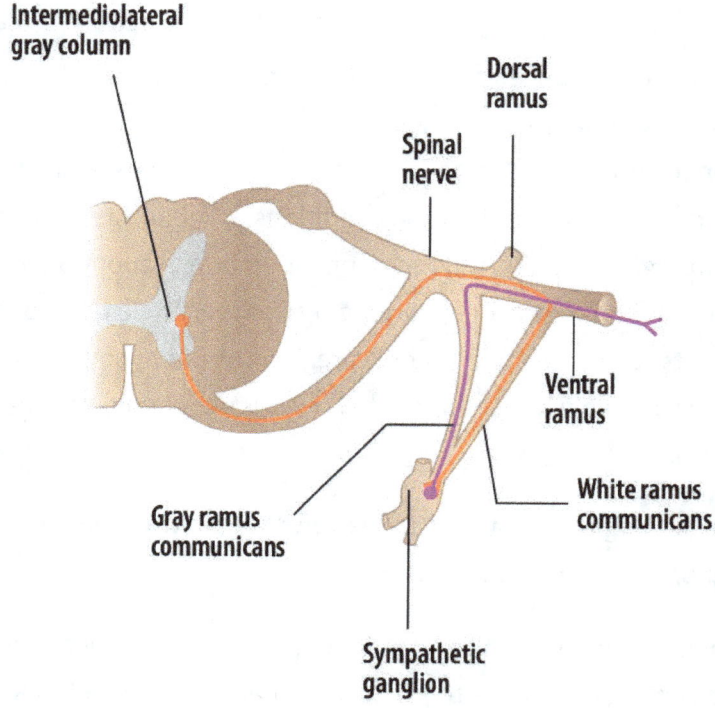

Intermediolateral gray column

Dorsal ramus

Spinal nerve

Ventral ramus

White ramus communicans

Gray ramus communicans

Sympathetic ganglion

Figure 3-4. Anatomy of the spinal cord, showing the location of the sympathetic nerves.

The combination of low blood pressure and low cardiac output significantly decreases the placenta's perfusion, leading to diminished oxygen delivery to the fetus. Fetal hypoxemia is often manifested as fetal heart bradycardia and systemic acidosis (fetal distress). This is manifested as a late deceleration of fetal heart rate with a loss of beat-to-beat variability, often referred to as an "ominous pattern" in fetal heart rate monitoring (Figure 3-5).

The epidural will also cause relaxed lower abdominal muscles. A patient lying on her back with these relaxed lower abdominal muscles can cause the gravid (or pregnant) uterus to rest on the abdominal aorta and the inferior vena cava (a condition called aortocaval compression syndrome), further compromising placental perfusion and fetal oxygenation.

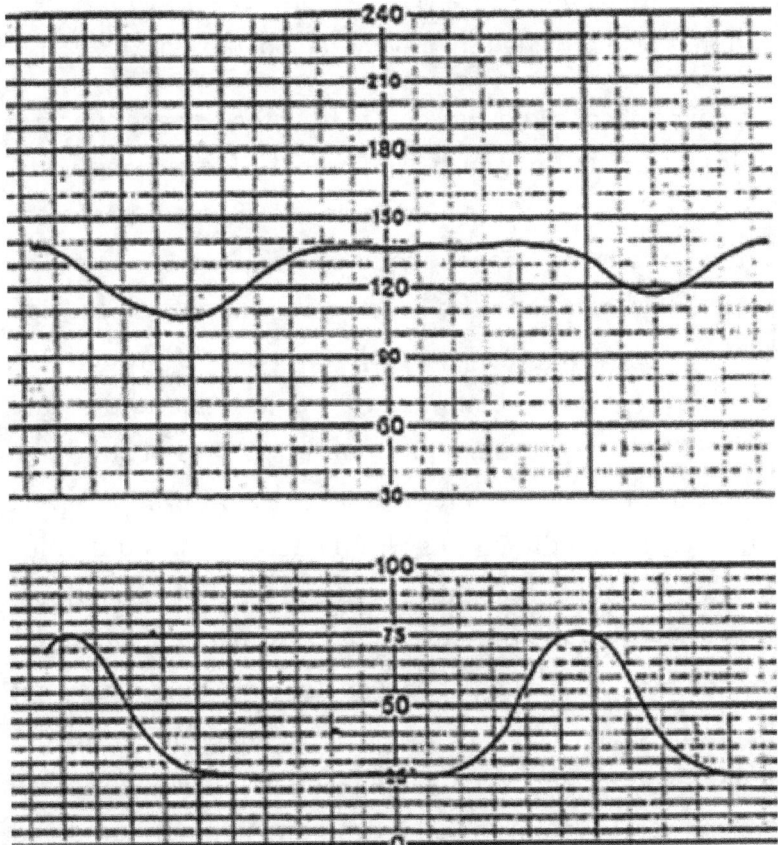

Figure 3-5. The graph shows a decrease in fetal heart rate (top) with each contraction of the uterus (bottom). Late decelerations are delayed with respect to the contraction of the uterus.

Anesthesiologists often anticipate a decrease in blood pressure and heart rate following the initiation of an epidural or spinal block, and they are well-trained in how to manage the potential adverse effects. For instance, to unload the aorta and vena cava from the pressing gravid uterus, they know to tilt the patient's pelvis to the left. The sympathectomy is treated with IV fluid bolus or medicines such as epinephrine, ephedrine, or phenylephrine. The slowed heart rate is restored with atropine or glycopyrrolate. Oxygen supplementation is also provided to prevent fetal hypoxemia.

However, despite knowing how to treat the adverse effects of epidurals, conditions such as maternal hypotension, bradycardia, fetal hypoxia, and fetal acidosis often occur, and the interventions may be inadequate or applied too late. The anesthesiologist and the nursing staff might not be vigilant in monitoring the potential occurrence of hypotension or bradycardia in the mother via frequent blood pressure checks following the epidural initiation. The obstetrician might not be comfortable with fetal scalp pH monitoring. There might be difficulties with IV access and fluid bolus administration. Resuscitative medications such as epinephrine, ephedrine, or atropine might not be readily available for immediate use. Oxygen or oxygen delivery sources may not be in the room. Time is of the essence, and minutes count if fetal hypoxia and brain damage are to be avoided. These "micro-hemodynamic instabilities," often unmonitored and inadequately treated, may play a significant role in the development of neuropsychiatric disorders in the newborn.

Another important contributing factor to the causation of fetal hypoxia by the epidural is the prolongation of both stage one and stage two labor. To avoid operative delivery, most obstetricians will start any infusion of oxytocin. Let's break down why this might contribute to fetal hypoxia.

To start with, when given an epidural, a woman experiences profound relaxation of the lower abdominal and pelvic muscles, which invariably leads to delays in the descent of the fetal head, leading to prolongation of stage one labor. The mother's inability to strain and push due to weakened muscles could very well lead to a more prolonged second stage of labor. An old obstetrical adage states, "No laboring mother should see more than one sunrise or sunset!" meaning that her labor should not last more than a full day. To this end, most obstetricians will use oxytocin to attempt to move labor that has slowed following an epidural. Starting oxytocin infusion after an epidural is now the standard of care. Powerful contractions triggered by oxytocin tend to counteract the delay caused by the epidural, so it is effective in getting labor to quicken.

Unfortunately, solid studies now show the worst outcomes for neurodevelopmental disorders when oxytocin is given to laboring mothers who are under epidural analgesia. A recent cohort study from California not only confirmed the association between autism and epidurals but also noted that the risk increased significantly when oxytocin was added to the therapeutic mix [26]. I believe this is because excessively strong muscular contractions initiated by oxytocin can impair circulation to the placenta, compromising fetal brain oxygenation.

To date, I'm not aware of any study that has investigated the occurrence of maternal hypotension, bradycardia, fetal brady-cardia, fetal acidosis, and the use of resuscitative medications during labor following the initiation of epidurals and the occurrence of developmental disabilities, including ASD. It is likely that a carefully conducted study that measures the area under the curve of fetal heart rate tracing will likely show significant fetal hypoxia in children who go on to develop autism. Nevertheless, well-designed studies are showing low Apgar scores, fetal hypoxia, and admission to the neonatal intensive care unit in neonates of low-risk women receiving epidural analgesia during birth [27].

It is my opinion that future studies will likely find a link between the use of epidurals and the occurrence of fetal brain hypoxemia and the increased incidence of ASD. It's essential to bear in mind that similar regions of the brain are damaged following mild to moderate hypoxemia and the pathology seen in ASD. Highly oxygen-sensitive regions of the brain—the hippocampus, amygdala, basal ganglia, cerebellum, and certain regions of the cerebral cortex—are often preferentially damaged by nonlethal hypoxemia, and these sites have been noted to be abnormal in children with ASD as well.

Additionally, it is likely that there is a relationship between ASD and ADHD. Both conditions involve early brain development issues and may result from similar mechanisms, such as oxygen deprivation or disrupted hormone signaling. They are both neurodevelopmental disorders characterized by onset in the early development period and deficits in several functional domains.

The Centers for Disease Control and Prevention indicates that 1 in 36 children in the United States is affected by ASD. Both disorders probably share the same mechanisms of brain injury, which results in a spectrum of deficiencies based on the severity of neuronal damage. Studies show that 15 to 25 percent of youth with ADHD meet the criteria for ASD, whereas 50 to 70 percent of those with ASD also have ADHD. The close association between the two disorders suggests a shared etiology and pathophysiology for both disorders.

Retrospective Studies of Offspring of Women Who Received Oxytocin

It's like peanut butter and jelly on toast—epidurals and oxytocin just go together. In most hospitals, as soon as the epidural catheter is placed, most obstetricians will order an IV infusion of oxytocin. The current practice advisory recommends oxytocin in all women receiving epidurals to reduce the rate of operative deliveries [28]. The epidural masks the strong contractions produced by the synthetic oxytocin, and oxytocin mitigates any slowing in the progression of the first stage of labor caused by the epidural. Thus, in most epidemiological studies, it's difficult to tease out whether it's the epidural causing autism or the synthetic oxytocin that's contributing to it. Yet, studies that have successfully isolated synthetic oxytocin as a single variable show a shockingly high incidence of autism in male offspring (incidence rates of 103.2 and 81.4 per 100,000 person-years, respectively) whose mothers' labors were augmented with synthetic oxytocin [29, 30].

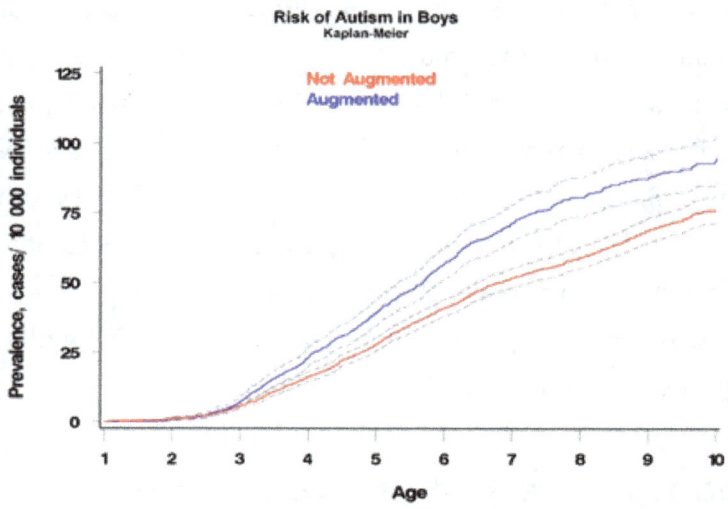

Figure 3-6. Autism risk in boys born to mothers who received oxytocin infusion.

In the majority of women, the epidural is the reason for oxytocin therapy. Without an epidural, rarely is there a need for oxytocin therapy. There is a causal connection between epidural and the adverse effects of oxytocin on the offspring. Oxytocin is a peptide hormone synthesized by the hypothalamus in the brain; then, it is transported to the posterior pituitary gland and released from there when needed. Naturally produced oxytocin is responsible for uterine contractions during labor and the ejection of milk from the breasts. In addition to these two primary functions, proper concentrations of naturally occurring oxytocin are responsible for mother-infant bonding, social attachment behaviors, empathy, reward, cognition, and creating a sense of calm and well-being [31, 32]. Several studies have shown low concentrations of naturally occurring oxytocin in children with ASD long after birth.

The epidural analgesia by itself diminishes endogenous oxytocin production in the mother [33]. The infusion of synthetic oxytocin makes things worse. The synthetic oxytocin administered peripherally has poor penetration through the blood-brain barrier. Yet, blasting the mother and the fetus with synthetic oxytocin several folds the natural levels of oxytocin [34] could turn off the production of natural oxytocin and irreparably harm the oxytocin receptor in the brain and elsewhere.

This is no different from what we observed in clinical practice with the use of corticosteroids to treat bronchial asthma or autoimmune diseases. After prolonged use of prednisone for treatment, the body loses its ability to produce intrinsic corticosteroids. This feedback inhibition of hormone secretion is also observed with other hormones like thyroxine and testosterone. There's no reason to believe oxytocin administration would behave any differently. Of the more than 963 genes related to the secretion and expression of oxytocin and its receptors, many are either turned off, downregulated, or permanently mutated by exposure to high concentrations of synthetic oxytocin at birth.

There are other immediate adverse effects of excessive synthetic oxytocin, both on the mother and the fetus during labor [35]. These include hyperstimulation of the uterus, resulting in uteroplacental insufficiency and diminished oxygen supply to the fetal brain. Excessive fluid retention due to oxytocin can lead to water intoxication and seizures in the mother, as well as tumultuous labor, uterine rupture, and cervical and vaginal tears. In the fetus, heart deceleration, hypoxia, hypercarbia, acidosis, and death have been reported with oxytocin infusion.

In summary, there's a strong correlation between the use of epidurals and the occurrence of ASD in children. Currently, scientists are not clear on the exact source of the cause, although it's highly likely a combination of factors, including microhemodynamic instabilities in the mother, toxicity of the local anesthetics, and frequent use of oxytocin augmentation of labor following epidurals, may all play a synergistic role in precipitating ASD in genetically vulnerable children.

Ultimately, when one looks at the prevalence of ASD and the use of epidurals by women of childbearing age, it becomes abundantly clear that the regions of the world where epidural analgesia is widely used are also the regions of high prevalence of ASD (Figure 3-1), leading one to conclude that there is a strong correlation between the two.

While we spent much of this chapter exploring the potential adverse effects of the epidural, it still may be the right choice for many expectant mothers. That being said, many other pain management options exist. In the next chapter, we'll explore an alternative to the epidural: spinal analgesia.

Chapter 4

SPINAL ANALGESIA

Spinal analgesia is an effective pain relief option to consider as an alternative to epidural anesthesia, particularly for women in the later stages of labor. It is quicker to administer and provides dense, predictable pain relief without the patchy effects that can sometimes occur with epidural blocks.

Spinal analgesia, also known as a subarachnoid block, involves injecting a local anesthetic into the subarachnoid space of the spine, which contains cerebrospinal fluid. This allows the anesthetic to mix with the cerebrospinal fluid, enabling it to ascend, descend, or remain at the injection level based on the density of the anesthetic used. The spinal block can be delivered as a single injection or continuously through a catheter placed in the subarachnoid space.

How the Spinal Is Performed

As shown in Figure 4-1, both spinal and epidural procedures are performed at the lumbar spine level. The patient can be sitting up or lying on her side, curled up in a fetal position. In an epidural, the tip of the spinal needle is placed outside the membrane that covers the spinal cord, known as the dura mater. There is no cerebrospinal fluid present in the epidural space. After placing the needle, an epidural catheter is inserted and left in the epidural space. Local anesthetics are then injected through the catheter into this area.

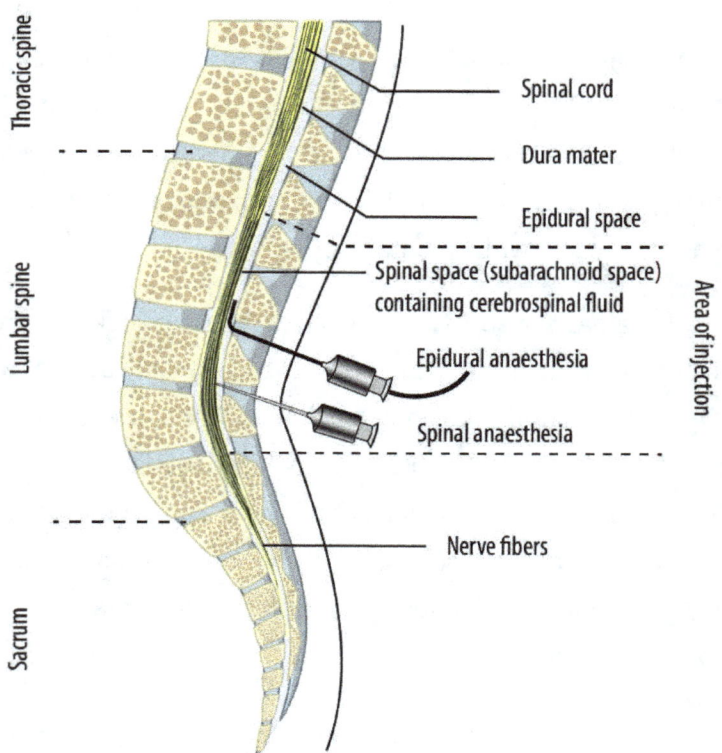

Figure 4-1. Anatomy of the spinal epidural and subarachnoid spaces.

These local anesthetics are believed to work by blocking nerve conduction at the level of the nerve roots within the spinal canal. In contrast, during a spinal procedure, the needle is advanced beyond the epidural space, through the dura mater, the arachnoid mater, and into the subarachnoid space, which contains cerebrospinal fluid. Spinal analgesia is known by different names in clinical practice, as listed in Figure 4-2. These names include spinal anesthesia, intrathecal block, subarachnoid block, "single shot," continuous spinal, and saddle block—all referring to the injection of local anesthetic into the spinal cerebrospinal fluid. The outflow of cerebrospinal fluid is a confirmatory sign that the needle is correctly positioned.

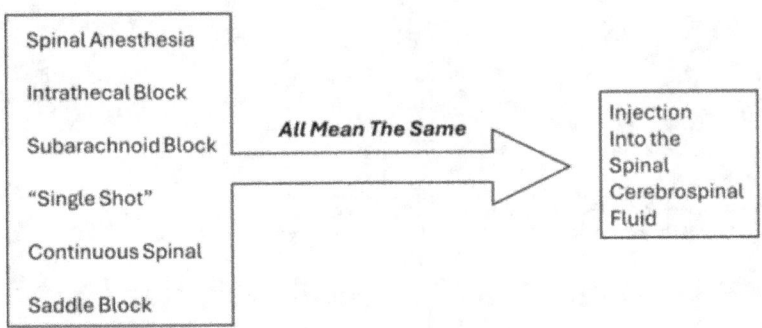

Spinal Anesthesia

Intrathecal Block

Subarachnoid Block

"Single Shot"

Continuous Spinal

Saddle Block

All Mean The Same

Injection Into the Spinal Cerebrospinal Fluid

Figure 4-2. Commonly used synonyms for spinal analgesia.

Local anesthetics injected into the subarachnoid space can either rise or descend based on the density of the local anesthetic solution compared to the density of the cerebrospinal fluid. Most anesthesiologists use a formulation that prevents the local anesthetic from ascending to higher thoracic and cervical regions. Accidental high levels of spinal analgesia can result in a very slow heart rate, a drop in blood pressure, and difficulty breathing. This occurs due to blockage of the sympathetic nervous system, which originates primarily from the T1 to L2 spinal segments, along with paralysis of the intercostal nerves arising from the T1 to T11 spinal cord segments.

As with epidural infusions, opioids such as fentanyl or morphine can be mixed with the local anesthetic and injected into the subarachnoid space. Opioid medications increase the analgesic density and duration of the spinal injection. Figure 4-3 gives an overview of the most commonly used medications in a spinal.

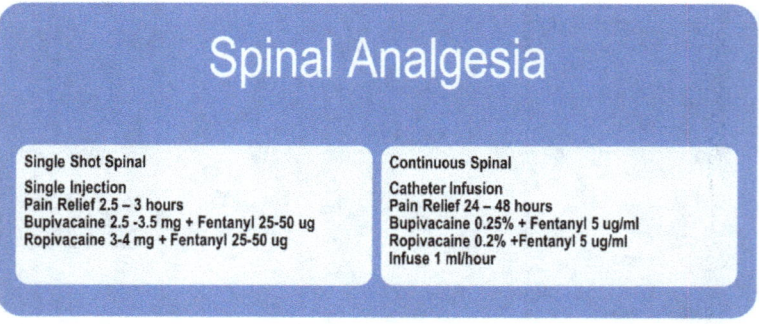

Figure 4-3. Commonly used medications in spinal analgesia.

As I mentioned in the previous section, spinal analgesia can be a single injection ("single shot") or a continuous infusion ("continuous spinal"). The single-shot injections are easy to perform and often take no more than 10 to 20 minutes to achieve good pain relief. Depending on the dosage of local anesthetic used, pain relief can last up to three hours, with the hope that the baby will be delivered by then. Otherwise, the injection may have to be repeated.

The other option is to insert a catheter and administer a continuous infusion of local anesthetics. Continuous spinal administration offers the advantage of prolonged pain relief and can be easily converted to spinal anesthesia if a C-section becomes necessary. This approach is particularly beneficial in specific clinical situations where predictable analgesia is needed and precise control of the anesthetic level is essential, such as in patients with edema, morbid obesity, or challenging airway conditions. The continuous spinal technique allows for administering small amounts of local anesthetics while monitoring the patient's spinal and hemodynamic stability closely. This method can be lifesaving for patients with compromised pulmonary function and difficult airways, as a high spinal may lead to severe complications, including failed airway management and even death. We will explore this scenario in the case study at the end of this chapter.

Complications of Spinal Analgesia

All of the complications we discussed in the previous chapter that relate to epidural analgesia are also common under spinal analgesia. Clinically, the most profound adverse effect is the sudden decrease in blood pressure and heart rate. If not immediately recognized and treated, this could lead to cardiac arrest and death. The sudden decrease in blood pressure and heart rate results from local anesthetics rising higher in the spinal cerebrospinal fluid and anesthetizing the sympathetic nervous system, which originates from the intermediolateral cell column of the spinal cord.

And, as we will see in the following case study, "total spinal" is also a serious risk with spinal analgesia, where the injected local anesthetic blocks the entire spinal cord. This is a catastrophic emergency, paralyzing the patient's respiratory muscles, heart, and blood vessels. The patient's trachea must be immediately intubated with a breathing tube, and positive pressure ventilation must be started. Epinephrine or other inotropic medications must be administered immediately to correct the drop in blood pressure and heart rate. Failure to intervene in a timely fashion will result in the death of the mother and possibly the loss of the baby.

Case Study: Deadly Complication of "Total Spinal"

The following facts are summarized from the New York Department of Health findings of fact in the case of *In the Matter of Dmitry Anatolevich Shelchkov, M.D.*, dated November 1, 2021.

Sha-Asia Semple was a 26-year-old pregnant patient who was 40 weeks and five days along when she came under the care of Dr. Dmitry Shelchkov at Woodhull Medical Center on July 3, 2020. Dr. Shelchkov administered a test dose of epidural anesthesia using lidocaine with epinephrine and fentanyl. Shortly after the procedure, the patient became anxious and reported difficulty breathing, saying, "I can't breathe; I feel funny," before becoming unresponsive. Despite resuscitation efforts, including intubation, she died two hours later.

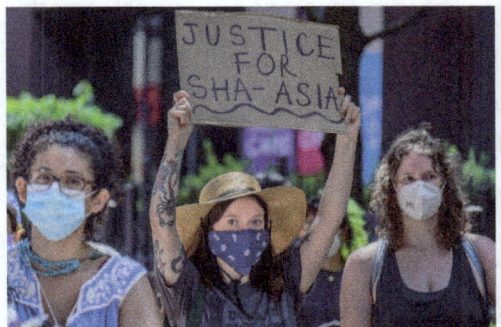 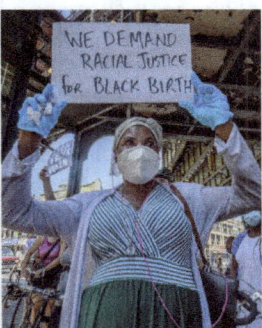

Figure 4-4. Sha-Asia Semple's death from total spinal sparked protests across New York City. Many women were unaware of this complication from epidural. (Copyright 2020 Alamy Inc.)

An autopsy revealed that the epidural catheter had been placed 34 centimeters deep into the subarachnoid space, leading to a total spinal—a condition where anesthetic drugs enter the central nervous system, suppressing respiration and resulting in acute hypoxic brain damage. The toxicology report indicated the presence of bupivacaine, a long-acting anesthetic, in her heart blood.

While it may be easy to find fault with Dr. Shelchkov for this tragic outcome, it's important to recognize the challenges he faced. In obese patients with moderate edema in the back, maneuvering the needle through a half-centimeter intervertebral space can be extremely difficult, especially without the aid of X-rays. The situation is further complicated when the anesthesiologist is called late in stage one of labor, during which contractions are strong and frequent. Patients often move, scream, cry, or seek comfort from others, making the spine a moving target. Under these conditions, placing the needle tip deep within the epidural space, rather than into the intrathecal space, is only a matter of a one-to-two-millimeter difference in depth. Understanding the anatomy of the spinal meninges (the membranous coverings of the spinal cord) highlights the difficulty of this task. Such mistakes can occur even for the most skilled and experienced anesthesiologists.

Unfortunately, Dr. Shelchkov failed to recognize the complication of injecting local anesthetic into the cerebrospinal fluid instead of the epidural space and did not take appropriate corrective action. The moral of the story is that "total spinals" are a real risk associated with epidural or spinal analgesia, and this potentially fatal risk is seldom communicated to patients during labor.

In the next chapter, we will look at some intravenous pain medications. We'll discuss how they can be used alone as patient-controlled analgesia (PCA) or as adjuncts to an epidural or spinal. We will also examine their side effects, particularly their ability to cross the placental barrier and cause sedation in the fetus.

Chapter 5

INTRAVENOUS ANALGESIA

Not every mother requires an epidural during childbirth. If you have a high pain tolerance or have already given birth to three or more children, you may not need any spinal intervention. However, this does not mean you won't need any pain relief at all. In fact, you might still benefit from some form of analgesia to help manage the pain and make it more tolerable. This is where intravenous pain medications can play an important role for women who prefer not to have epidurals, spinals, or nerve blocks during labor.

While intravenous medications may not be as effective as epidurals in controlling labor pain, they provide moderate relief and can reduce the intensity of strong uterine contractions. Opioid medications, which have been used for centuries, are known to deliver excellent pain relief during the early stages of labor. They can also be used alongside other pain relief methods, including epidurals. Even women who choose natural childbirth may find that small doses of opioid injections in the later stages of the first phase of labor are beneficial.

One significant advantage of opioids is that their side effects can be quickly reversed with an antidote called naloxone. If a baby appears lethargic or does not breathe or cry vigorously after the mother has received opioids for pain management, administering a small amount of naloxone—either as a nasal drop or as an intramuscular or intravenous injection—can rapidly restore the infant's alertness and breathing.

The common opioids used to provide labor analgesia in the United States are shown in Table 5-1. While opioids are typically administered intravenously (via an IV) for immediate pain relief, they can also be given as intramuscular injections (IM). Although the peak effect of IM injections is delayed, the pain relief they provide lasts longer.

OPIOID	DOSE	ONSET	DURATION	REPEAT
Morphine	5 mg (IV) 10 mg (IM)	5 min. 30 min.	1-2 hrs. 2-4 hrs.	Q 2 hrs. Q 4 hrs.
Meperidine	50 mg (IV) 100 mg (IM)	5 min. 30 min.	1-2 hrs. 2-4 hrs.	Q 2 hrs. Q 4 hrs.
Fentanyl	50-75 ug (IV)	1 min.	45 min.	Q 1 hr.
Stadol	2 mg	2 min. (IV) 20 min. (IM)	1-2 hrs. 2-4 hrs.	Q 2 hrs. Q 4 hrs.
Nubain	10 mg	3 min. (IV) 15 min. (IM)	1-2 hrs. 2-3 hrs.	Q 3 hrs. Q 4 hrs.

Table 5-1. Commonly used opioids in labor analgesia.

Patient Controlled Analgesia

Current literature suggests that administering short-acting remifentanil through intravenous patient-controlled analgesia (PCA) is one of the most effective methods for managing pain in parturients who either prefer not to receive or cannot have spinal neuraxial analgesia.

PCA allows patients to self-administer pain medication by pressing a button that activates an IV infusion pump containing the medication. This system enables patients to avoid waiting for a nurse to provide pain relief. The physician programs the infusion pump to deliver a predetermined dose each time the button is pressed. For safety reasons, a maximum amount of medication that can be dispensed within a specific timeframe, known as a lockout interval, is also established. This precaution helps prevent overdosing.

Research indicates that PCA therapy allows patients to achieve optimal pain relief with minimal sedation and fewer side effects. Remifentanil IV-PCA is typically administered at a dose of 20 to 60 micrograms per bolus, with a lockout interval of two minutes. The drug is highly effective—nearly 100 times more potent than morphine—with effects that begin within two to four minutes and last for 10 to 20 minutes. Therefore, it is best delivered as an infusion, as turning off the infusion allows for rapid recovery.

However, at higher doses, remifentanil can cause respiratory depression and severe bradycardia in the mother. Additionally, it crosses the placenta into the fetal circulation, which may slow the fetal heart rate. Fortunately, the incidence of this adverse effect is minimal when remifentanil is administered within the recommended dose range.

Extra vigilance is necessary after the baby is born to reverse any residual effects of the opioid on the baby, such as a slow heart rate and depressed respiration. If the baby appears sedated, with depressed breathing, then an opioid reversal agent such as naloxone should be administered to the baby without wasting time. The response to naloxone is often quick and dramatic and will save the baby from endotracheal intubation and mechanical ventilation.

Several other anesthetic agents are currently being tried for labor analgesia. Two of them, ketamine and dexmedetomidine, hold the promise of offering real alternatives to opioid medications.

Ketamine is a powerful dissociative anesthetic agent. At higher doses, it causes general anesthesia. At lower doses, it can be used as an analgesic. Unlike opioid medications, ketamine has minimal adverse effects on the mother's blood pressure, heart rate, and respiration. A low-dose ketamine infusion (loading dose of 0.2 mg/kg delivered over 30 minutes, followed by an infusion at 0.2 mg/kg/hr) can provide adequate analgesia during labor and delivery. In clinical trials, maternal blood flow and fetal heart rate were not affected by ketamine infusion [36].

Dexmedetomidine is an alpha-2 adrenergic agonist with profound sedative and analgesic effects. It can cause slowing of the heart and depression of respiration. In lower doses, in addition to its ability to deepen the analgesic effects of local anesthetics when used as an adjunct in labor epidurals, the intravenous administration can provide satisfactory analgesia in many laboring women. Notably, while pain relief with the administration of dexmedetomidine was adequate, most of the patients became deeply sedated as well. A 1 ug/kg bolus followed by an infusion of 0.2–1.0 ug/kg/hr dexmedetomidine provides excellent pain relief for phases one and two of labor [37].

Complications

Intravenous analgesics present a compelling alternative to epidurals for managing pain during labor. They can be administered quickly, and with careful dosage adjustments, they provide effective pain relief. However, there are risks associated with their use. These include potential depression of cardiovascular functions, such as heart rate and blood pressure, as well as respiratory suppression, which could lead to respiratory arrest if the patient is not closely monitored.

Another concern is excessive sedation, particularly for parturients who may require higher doses of opioids for adequate pain relief. Some opioids, like morphine and fentanyl, can trigger the release of histamine from mast cells, resulting in transient itching and wheezing. It is crucial to note that all intravenously administered medications can cross the placenta and potentially affect the fetus. In significant amounts, they may depress fetal heart function, inhibit spontaneous respiration, and cause sedation in the newborn. If higher doses are used or if the medication is administered over an extended period, staff trained in neonatal resuscitation should be present at the time of delivery, prepared to intervene if necessary.

In the next chapter, we will explore general anesthesia, an extreme form of pain relief. Although it is highly effective, it is rarely used during normal labor. We will closely examine both the advantages and disadvantages of general anesthesia in mitigating labor pain.

Chapter 6

GENERAL ANESTHESIA FOR LABOR

General anesthesia is an option to consider for managing labor pain in certain situations. While it is effective for pain relief, it requires careful consideration due to potential complications. General anesthetic agents can be divided into two categories: (1) intravenous anesthetics, such as sodium thiopental and propofol, and (2) inhalation agents, including nitrous oxide and various forms of ethers like halothane, isoflurane, sevoflurane, and desflurane.

Among these categories, intravenous agents should not be used for labor analgesia because the risks significantly outweigh the benefits. In contrast, inhalation agents can be used during labor to provide effective pain relief. This chapter will focus on inhalation anesthesia for managing labor pain.

Inhalation Ethers

In lower doses, inhalation anesthetics such as halothane, isoflurane, sevoflurane, and desflurane can provide significant pain relief without inducing loss of consciousness. However, there are two major disadvantages associated with their use:

1. They cause dose-dependent relaxation of the uterine muscles, which can halt the expulsion of the fetus and stop the progression of labor.

2. Analgesia can imperceptibly transition into general anesthesia.

These anesthetic agents can easily cross the placenta and reach the fetal brain in concentrations sufficient to anesthetize both the fetus and the mother. Babies born to mothers who have received general anesthesia often appear sedated and limp, showing weak activity, diminished crying, and a depressed heart rate. Until the anesthetics are eliminated from the infant's system, they may require assisted breathing and intravenous fluids.

Because of the potential for profound uterine relaxation and labor arrest with the induction of general anesthesia, inhalation anesthetics are rarely used in modern obstetrics. When used for analgesia, these agents must be administered intermittently, similar to nitrous oxide, during contractions.

Furthermore, many anesthesia providers lack the training or competence to carry out this approach effectively. There is ongoing concern that inhalation analgesia could inadvertently shift into deeper levels of anesthesia, even in well-trained hands. With the initiation of anesthesia, there is a genuine risk that the laboring individual could become unconscious, lose the ability to breathe, and be unable to protect their lungs from aspirating gastric contents.

In addition, these inhalation agents are highly lipid-soluble and diffuse quickly across the placenta, often resulting in the baby being anesthetized. If prompt assistance is not available for resuscitating the baby, serious harm can occur due to insufficient oxygen reaching the brain.

Despite these drawbacks, inhalation anesthetics may be necessary in cases of acute fetal distress during the latter half of the second stage of labor. In such situations, forceps or vaginal operative delivery may be the only means to safely expedite the delivery of a stuck baby when it may be too late to consider spinal or epidural analgesia.

In these circumstances, the continuous administration of inhalation agents provides rapid pain relief and sufficient uterine relaxation, which facilitates the vaginal delivery of the baby. In the third stage of labor, after the baby is delivered, the entire placenta or fragments of it may remain stuck in the uterus. This can prevent the uterus from fully contracting, leading to ongoing bleeding. The obstetrician may need to insert a hand or instruments into the uterus to remove the retained products of conception. Inhalation agents can provide adequate uterine relaxation and pain relief to assist the obstetrician in completing this task.

Under these conditions, the anesthesia provider must be prepared to manage the potential loss of consciousness in the mother. This may involve performing effective mask ventilation and, if necessary, intubating the trachea with a cuffed endotracheal tube to protect the airways from aspiration and ensure adequate positive pressure ventilation of the lungs.

In modern obstetrics, the use of inhalational general anesthetics for vaginal delivery should be rare. With proper prenatal examinations and ultrasound measurements, most of these patients should be counseled to consider an elective cesarean section.

Nitrous Oxide

Among all general anesthetic agents, nitrous oxide (N_2O) has the fewest adverse effects on both the mother and the baby. Due to its low lipid solubility, nitrous oxide rapidly reaches therapeutic levels, providing moderate pain relief with minimal impact on the fetus.

For it to be effective, the gas should be inhaled at the onset of a contraction and continued throughout the contraction, stopping as soon as the contraction ends. This method of intermittent administration minimizes the risk of hypoxia in the mother while offering sufficient pain relief to alleviate the peak pain associated with contractions (Figure 6-1).

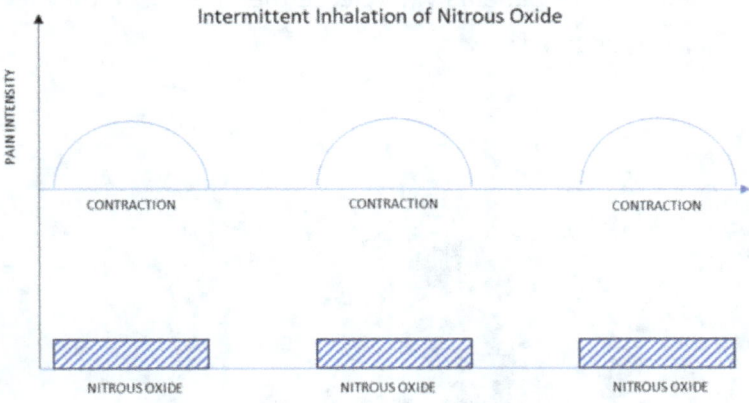

Figure 6-1. Intermittent administration of nitrous oxide. Breathing coincides with uterine contractions.

In one study [38] involving 1,958 parturients, the investigators found a satisfaction score of 7.4 out of 10 in women who used nitrous oxide for pain relief. However, nearly two-thirds of the women went on to request an epidural for their pain relief due to inadequate pain relief from nitrous oxide.

In my opinion, while this option may be adequate for some women, nitrous oxide alone has been shown to be insufficient to provide satisfactory pain relief in women having their first or second baby. In combination with intravenous opioids, however, nitrous oxide can provide significant pain relief.

Nitrous oxide is mixed with oxygen to create 50 percent, 60 percent, or 70 percent nitrous oxide concentrations to prevent hypoxemia. Patients self-administer the gas using a mouthpiece or face mask (see Figure 6-2). This method, where the patient holds the mask, helps minimize the risk of overdose and excessive sedation, as patients will release the mask once they feel sufficiently sedated.

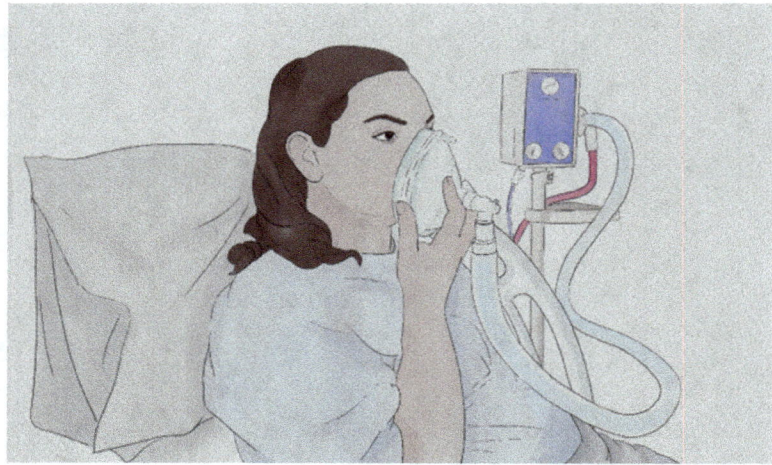

Figure 6-2. Nitrous oxide is often self-administered. This prevents overdose and hypoxia.

The American College of Obstetricians and Gynecologists advises against combining sedatives and hypnotics with nitrous oxide administration due to the risk of hypoxia in mothers. However, small doses of intravenous opioids can enhance the analgesic effects of nitrous oxide and help avoid hypoxemia in well-monitored hospital settings.

For optimal effectiveness, nitrous oxide inhalation should begin 20 to 30 seconds before contractions start and continue throughout the contraction. The best results occur when the mother takes four deep breaths initially to saturate her lungs and then breathes normally during the contractions. It is generally recommended not to inhale nitrous oxide between contractions, as this may increase the risk of hypoxia and cause altered mentation. Inhalation of nitrous oxide can be combined with intravenous opioids, such as Demerol, to achieve a satisfactory level of analgesia. Additionally, other potent analgesics, like ketamine, can provide effective pain relief in small doses when used as adjuncts to nitrous oxide inhalation.

In summary, inhaling nitrous oxide is a suitable option for mothers who prefer not to use spinal or epidural analgesia during labor. Nitrous oxide can be effectively combined with intravenous opioids or low-dose ketamine to offer satisfactory pain relief. Additionally, other inhalation anesthetics may provide effective analgesia in situations where the baby's head is stuck at the vaginal outlet, and fetal distress is imminent. These anesthetics also ensure adequate uterine relaxation and pain relief during the extraction of retained placenta.

In the next chapter, we will explore the different anesthetic options available for cesarean delivery. If a patient already has an epidural or intrathecal spinal catheter in place for pain relief, it will be straightforward to use the same catheter for spinal anesthesia. If not, we may need to perform spinal or epidural anesthesia, or in some cases, general anesthesia may be necessary. We will discuss the advantages and disadvantages of each anesthetic method.

Chapter 7

ANESTHESIA FOR CESAREAN DELIVERY

Every pregnant woman, whether or not she has planned for it, should be psychologically prepared for the possibility of a cesarean delivery, commonly referred to as a C-section.

A cesarean delivery involves the surgeon making a horizontal incision in the lower abdomen to access the uterus. The lower part of the uterus is then incised, allowing for the manual extraction of the baby. Cesarean deliveries are performed when vaginal delivery is not feasible or poses significant risks to either the mother or the baby.

Many C-sections are elective and can be scheduled months before the expected due date. However, some are urgent, occurring soon after a failed labor attempt, while others require immediate surgical intervention to save the life of the mother or the baby. Common reasons for cesarean deliveries fall into these three categories, as outlined in Table 7-1.

Elective	Urgent	STAT/Emergent
Cephalopelvic disproportion	Failure of labor to progress	Uterine rupture
Multiple births	Diabetes	Placental abruption
Breech position	Preeclampsia	Severe fetal distress
Repeat cesarean	Fetal distress	Cord prolapse
Birth defects	Maternal exhaustion	Severe maternal distress
Fibroid uterus	Sepsis	Pulmonary embolism
Vaginal deformity		High spinal analgesia
Active vaginal herpes		
Placenta previa		

Table 7-1. Common causes of cesarean section.

All types of C-sections require anesthesia to ensure the safe delivery of the baby. The spinal analgesia used during the trial of labor is often not strong enough for patients to endure the pain associated with abdominal incisions and uterine manipulation. However, I have seen skilled surgeons successfully perform cesarean sections using only a local anesthetic before the abdominal incision. This approach should only be used in extreme circumstances, such as when expert anesthesia personnel or equipment are unavailable and there is an urgent need to save the mother or child.

In the United States, most cesarean sections are performed using spinal anesthesia. Unlike general anesthesia, this technique means that the baby is not significantly affected by anesthetic agents administered to the mother. With spinal anesthesia, the mother remains awake while her abdomen and lower limbs lose sensitivity to pain, touch, temperature, and motor control. The amount of local anesthetic injected into the spine is minimal, so only a tiny amount enters the bloodstream and crosses the placenta, which has a negligible effect on the baby.

In patients who already have an epidural in place, it is necessary to deepen the density of the block to allow for surgery. This is typically accomplished by injecting a higher concentration of local anesthetic through the existing epidural catheter. This technique achieves complete insensitivity and loss of motor control, akin to spinal anesthesia. Figure 7-1 illustrates the choice of anesthesia for cesarean sections.

Epidurals typically take considerable time to perform, usually between 30 to 45 minutes. This duration includes administering a test dose and giving a bolus dose to achieve an adequate level of anesthesia. In contrast, the induction of general anesthesia is much faster. The anesthetic agent is injected through an intravenous line, allowing surgical levels of anesthesia to be reached in only five to seven minutes.

This quick induction is a key reason why general anesthesia is often preferred for STAT and emergency cesarean sections. Spinal anesthesia takes about 15 to 20 minutes to perform and achieve the required surgical level of regional anesthesia.

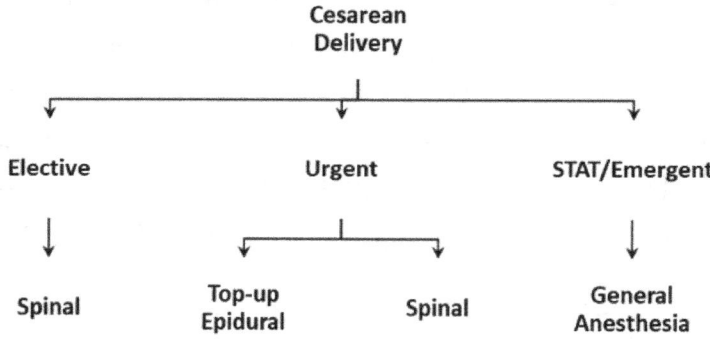

Figure 7-1. Anesthesia options for cesarean delivery.

In elective cases, where both the mother and baby are stable, there is no urgency, allowing the anesthesia provider to take the necessary time to administer an effective spinal block. In urgent situations, or if the epidural is ineffective, the provider may choose to perform a spinal anesthetic.

One advantage of spinal anesthesia is that it provides a dense surgical block while minimizing the amount of anesthetic agent that reaches the baby.

Risks of Anesthesia

All types of anesthesia come with certain risks that depend on the medication used, how it's given, and any preexisting health issues the patient may have, especially during labor. For example, spinal anesthesia may not cause a drop in blood pressure in patients who are well-hydrated. However, it can lead to dangerously low blood pressure in someone who is dehydrated due to not drinking enough fluids or not receiving enough intravenous fluids. Let's take a look at some of the possible complications associated with each type of anesthesia.

Immediate Complications of Spinal Anesthesia

Immediate complications from spinal anesthesia can occur within minutes of administration. The two most common and serious complications are sudden drops in blood pressure (hypotension) and excessive slowing of the heart rate (bradycardia). These issues arise because the local anesthetic injected into the spinal subarachnoid space paralyzes the sympathetic nervous system, which primarily regulates blood pressure and heart rate.

The sympathetic nervous system originates from the intermediolateral cell column of the spinal cord, specifically from the T1 to L2 segments. Consequently, higher doses of local anesthetic or a larger volume of spinal injectate can lead to a spinal blockade that ascends higher, potentially reaching the neck. When the spinal block is above the inter-nipple line (around T4), it is often associated with significant hypotension, bradycardia, and oxygen desaturation.

If left untreated, this can compromise blood flow to the placenta and reduce oxygen delivery to the fetus, resulting in hypoxic brain injury. Similarly, progressive hypotension and bradycardia can pose serious risks for the mother, potentially leading to severe brain injury or total cardiac arrest.

One critical lesson from analyzing the American Society of Anesthesiologists (ASA) closed legal claims database is the importance of early intervention when observing declines in blood pressure and heart rate post-spinal anesthesia. Medications like epinephrine, ephedrine, and phenylephrine can swiftly reverse falling blood pressure, while atropine or glycopyrrolate can be used to increase heart rate. An effective preventative measure is to administer 500 to 1,000 ml of IV fluid to the parturient 15 to 30 minutes prior to the planned spinal anesthesia. Additionally, tilting the patient's pelvis to the left with a foam wedge under the right buttocks (known as a left uterine tilt) can help relieve pressure on the inferior vena cava, enhancing venous return to the heart and helping maintain blood pressure and heart rate.

In rare instances, the spinal block can ascend to a level where the patient becomes completely numb from the neck down, a condition referred to as a "high spinal," which occurs above T4. This may paralyze the intercostal muscles, which are necessary for lung ventilation. Patients may occasionally report tingling or numbness in their fingers, which is a concerning sign indicating that the anesthetic is spreading to the cervical region of the spinal cord. In such cases, the anesthesiologist must provide supplemental oxygen and assist with ventilation using a face-mask and Ambu bag or a more invasive airway device. Airway management should occur concurrently with efforts to address the significant drops in blood pressure and heart rate that typically accompany a high spinal.

In rare and severe circumstances, the anesthetic may rise into the cervical region, causing paralysis of the upper extremities and the phrenic nerve, which controls the diaphragm. This condition, referred to as a "total spinal," can result in respiratory arrest and, if untreated, lead to cardiac arrest. Death can occur for both the mother and baby if not managed quickly, making prompt action critical. Blood pressure and heart rate must be treated immediately with the previously mentioned inotropic agents, and respiration must be supported with supplemental oxygen until the effects of the anesthetic wear off. It may also be necessary to induce general anesthesia, intubate the patient, and mechanically ventilate them until they regain spontaneous breathing. Death can often be avoided through timely assisted ventilation with supplemental oxygen and the administration of epinephrine or ephedrine to stabilize blood pressure and heart rate.

Aside from these serious complications, other immediate effects of spinal anesthesia include nausea and vomiting, which, although less serious, are more common. These symptoms can arise from various causes, including pressure on the stomach while lying flat on the operating table, which may lead to regurgitation and nausea. Other causes may involve signals from the brainstem due to inadequate oxygen, low blood pressure, or decreased heart rate. Administering supplemental oxygen and managing hypotension generally alleviates symptoms of nausea and vomiting promptly.

Delayed Complications of Spinal Anesthesia

When discussing delayed complications after a spinal injection, two complications are noteworthy: one is common, while the other is rare but can cause significant distress. The more common complication is known as a post-dural puncture headache (PDPH). This is an intense headache typically felt behind the eyes, on the sides of the head, and at the back of the head. It can occur minutes after the spinal injection or may appear several hours later, usually the next day, when the patient becomes more active after resting in bed following delivery.

A key feature of PDPH is its relationship to posture. The headache intensifies when sitting, standing, or walking and tends to lessen when the patient lies flat. This headache is believed to occur due to a decrease in cerebrospinal fluid (CSF) pressure inside the skull, which causes the brain and cranial nerves to sag, leading to pain. The CSF typically cushions the brain, but when a spinal needle punctures the dura mater, small amounts of fluid can leak into the epidural space, lowering CSF pressure.

Most cases of PDPH can be managed with time. Over 80 to 90 percent of patients find their headaches subside within five to seven days as the body heals the puncture in the dura mater. Recommended treatments include drinking plenty of fluids, taking oral non-steroidal anti-inflammatory drugs (NSAIDs), and staying flat in bed as much as possible.

In rare cases, if the headache severely limits activities or if it is accompanied by symptoms such as double vision, ringing in the ears, or nausea and vomiting, a more definitive treatment, called an "epidural blood patch," may be necessary. During this procedure, an anesthesiologist injects 10 to 20 ml of the patient's blood into the epidural space near where the spinal injection was performed. The blood clots and seals the hole in the dura, preventing further leakage of CSF. When done correctly, an epidural blood patch can provide immediate and lasting relief from PDPH. However, this procedure should be approached cautiously, as injected blood can lead to infections or adhesions in the epidural space.

The second delayed complication is less common but significant: lumbar nerve radiculopathy. Patients may experience pain, tingling, numbness, or weakness in one or both legs, which might occur if the spinal needle accidentally pierces a spinal nerve root or if the local anesthetic is injected into the nerve root. Fortunately, these symptoms typically resolve on their own over several months.

Often, these neurological injuries are more likely caused by the lithotomy position used during delivery rather than by the spinal needle itself. In the lithotomy position, the legs are raised and supported, which can stretch and potentially injure the nerve roots. Additionally, if the baby is particularly large, the nerve roots may become compressed between the baby's head and the pelvic bones. If symptoms are severe, a neurology consultation, lumbar spine MRI, and nerve conduction studies may be necessary. Usually, the best approach is to give it time, along with physiotherapy, for spontaneous recovery.

Epidural Anesthesia

Epidural anesthesia is often the preferred choice if a patient already has an epidural catheter in place for labor analgesia and a cesarean section is planned due to failure to progress or other maternal or fetal reasons. Regional anesthesia is achieved by injecting a higher concentration of local anesthetic, which creates a denser blockade of sensations and results in paralysis of motor functions. The complications associated with epidural anesthesia are similar to those of spinal anesthesia and include:

- Hypotension

- Bradycardia

- High spinal or total spinal anesthesia

- Post-dural puncture headache

- Permanent paresthesia in the lower limbs

Additionally, there are two complications that are somewhat unique to epidural anesthesia. The first is the risk of intravascular injection of a large volume of local anesthetic. Sometimes, the epidural catheter can inadvertently enter an epidural vein, functioning like an intravenous catheter. If the anesthesiologist fails to test for aspiration of blood from the catheter, a significant amount of local anesthetic could be injected intravenously. This may lead to local anesthetic systemic toxicity, where the patient typically experiences numbness and tingling in the lips, a metallic taste, and ringing in the ears. If these symptoms are not quickly recognized and the epidural infusion is not stopped, they can progress to muscle twitching in the limbs, cardiac arrhythmias, hypotension, and convulsions, potentially resulting in profound hypoxemia and cardiac arrest. It is essential for the physician to recognize this complication, provide supportive care, and administer intravenous 20 percent lipid emulsion, which can reverse the toxic effects of the local anesthetic. A careful anesthesiologist will always aspirate and then administer a small test dose before injecting a large amount of local anesthetic through the epidural catheter.

The second serious complication, which occurs more frequently after a spinal injection, is the development of an epidural hematoma. Since epidural needles are larger than spinal needles, the risk of trauma to the epidural plexus of veins is greater with the epidural technique. Furthermore, the insertion of the epidural catheter can cause additional bleeding from the epidural veins.

A slowly expanding hematoma in the epidural space can compress the spinal cord or the cauda equina, resulting in paralysis of the lower limbs and loss of bladder and bowel control. Patients may report tightness or aching pain in the lower spine, which may be masked by the local anesthetic. It can be several hours before weakness in the lower limbs and loss of bladder and bowel control become apparent. An immediate MRI of the spine is necessary to confirm the presence or absence of an epidural hematoma. If present, emergency spinal surgery must be performed to evacuate the hematoma and control the bleeding to prevent permanent paralysis.

This is a severe and devastating complication, and anesthesiologists must always consider it when performing a challenging epidural or spinal procedure, especially in patients with bleeding tendencies. In pregnancy, conditions such as HELLP syndrome (hemolysis, elevated liver enzymes, and low platelets) may lead to low platelet counts, increasing the risk of bleeding. In such cases, it is advisable to avoid epidural anesthesia or analgesia if the platelet count is below 100,000 per microliter of blood.

General Anesthesia

General anesthesia using inhalational anesthetic agents such as isoflurane, sevoflurane, or desflurane is typically reserved for urgent or emergency cesarean sections or instrumented vaginal deliveries. However, these agents have several significant disadvantages:

1. **Profound Uterine Relaxation.** These anesthetics can cause significant relaxation of the uterus, which may prevent it from contracting to expel the fetus. The labor comes to a halt. If the cervix is sufficiently dilated

and the fetal head is positioned at the perineum, the obstetrician may be able to perform a forceps delivery. Otherwise, a cesarean section will be necessary.

2. **Fetal Anesthesia.** The inhalational agents can cross the placenta and lead to general anesthesia in the fetus. As a result, newborns may be born fully anesthetized, necessitating expert medical intervention to support their breathing and maintain blood pressure.

3. **Maternal Loss of Consciousness.** Due to their potency, inhalational anesthetics can induce unconsciousness within just a few deep breaths. This loss of consciousness impairs the mother's ability to protect her airway and maintain spontaneous breathing, increasing the risk of aspirating acidic gastric contents into the lungs, which can lead to acute respiratory failure and even death. If the mother becomes unconscious, the anesthesiologist must quickly insert a cuffed breathing tube into the trachea to safeguard against aspiration and provide necessary ventilation. Aspiration of gastric contents is a leading cause of maternal mortality worldwide.

Despite these challenges, general anesthesia is often used in developing countries for instrumental vaginal delivery. The delivery should be ideally undertaken in the operating room, with instruments and anesthetics ready for a C-section. After the appropriate preparations for endotracheal intubation are complete, inhalational anesthetics like nitrous oxide can be administered intermittently through a mask during contractions, offering pain relief without significantly affecting uterine contractions. Most obstetricians will continue an oxytocin infusion at this stage.

When the fetal head has descended enough to allow for the application of forceps, inhalational agents may be administered continuously for deeper anesthesia. Typically, anesthesiologists will then deepen the anesthesia with intravenous agents such as barbiturates or propofol, followed by a muscle relaxant, and proceed with tracheal intubation. This approach helps to prevent aspiration of vomitus while ensuring proper ventilation and deeper anesthesia. The relaxation of the uterus and pelvic musculature can facilitate the application of forceps and the safe extraction of the fetal head.

Steps Involved In Emergency Cesarean Section

For those undergoing an emergency cesarean section, it can be helpful to know the steps involved in inducing general anesthesia. Familiarizing yourself with these steps can ease anxiety about the procedure. If you have specific requests, such as having your partner cut the umbilical cord or taking photographs during delivery, it's advisable to include them in your birth plan.

- **STEP 1**: Your anesthesia provider will assess your airway by looking into your mouth and evaluating the degree of mobility in your cervical spine. The provider will then make sure the appropriate instruments are available to secure your airway after you fall asleep.

- **STEP 2**: Your nursing staff will ensure you have a freely flowing IV.

- **STEP 3**: You will be given some form of nonparticulate antacid to neutralize the stomach acid.

- **STEP 4**: You will be taken to the operating room with continuous fetal heart rate monitoring.

- **STEP 5**: Once you're in the operating room, monitors will be applied to measure your vital signs while you're given 100 percent oxygen to breathe.

- **STEP 6**: A Foley catheter will be placed to empty your bladder.

- **STEP 7**: The operating room nurse will prep your abdomen with antiseptic and drape the abdomen with sterile fabric.

- **STEP 8**: One of the assistants will apply downward pressure to your neck (cricoid pressure) to prevent gastric content from regurgitating into your pharynx.

- **STEP 9**: The anesthesiologist will inject propofol (or another appropriate intravenous anesthetic), followed by a muscle relaxant such as rocuronium or succinylcholine. Going to sleep will be your last conscious experience until you wake up with a baby.

- **STEP 10**: After you're asleep, the anesthesiologist will perform an endotracheal intubation. This will prevent the aspiration of gastric content and provide a conduit for positive pressure ventilation.

- **STEP 11**: General anesthesia will be maintained by administering volatile agents through the breathing tube. Nitrous oxide and intravenous opioids, benzodiazepines, or antiemetics may be administered as part of a balanced anesthesia treatment.

- **STEP 12**: As soon as the endotracheal tube is in place, the obstetrician will make the abdominal incision and proceed to deliver the baby through an incision in the lower part of the uterus. Generally, time is of the essence when delivering distressed babies.

- **STEP 13**: Following the delivery of the baby and the placenta, if the uterus has not contracted sufficiently, then oxytocin bolus (20 units) followed by an infusion (20 units in 500 ml NS) will usually be started to promote uterine contraction and diminish bleeding.

- **STEP 14**: Once the skin closure is complete, all anesthetic agents will be turned off, and the patient will be allowed to breathe 100 percent oxygen. Any residual muscle relaxant will be reversed with suitable reversal agents.

- **STEP 15**: After a few minutes, the patient should resume breathing spontaneously and begin to awaken. Once the patient is responding to commands, the endotracheal tube will be removed.

- **STEP 16**: Once patients are stable, they will be transported back to the ward.

An in-depth discussion of the complications secondary to the C-section are beyond the scope of this text. However, it must be pointed out that time is critical when delivering babies in distress. The time from the initial skin incision to the uterine incision should not exceed five to eight minutes, and the time from the start of the uterine incision to the delivery of the baby should not exceed three to five minutes. Delays exceeding eight minutes from the skin incision to delivery are often linked to adverse fetal outcomes [39, 40].

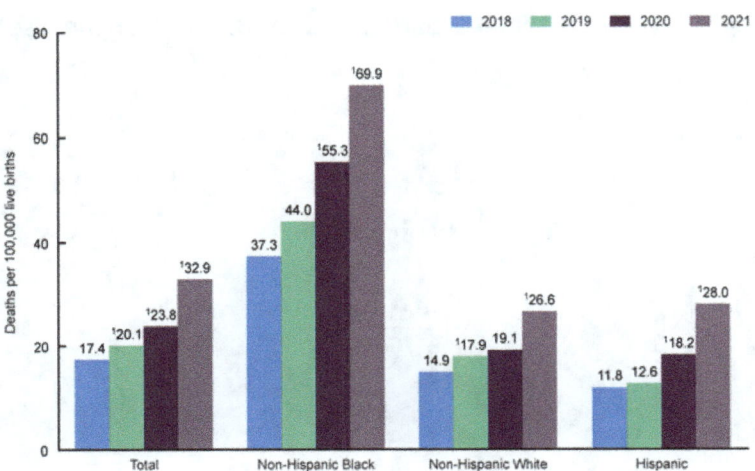

Figure 7-2. Maternal mortality by race in the US (2022).

Prolonged unnecessary actions, such as dissecting layers of tissues, cauterizing every bleeding vessel, applying and adjusting retractors, altering the lighting, or shifting the operating table, can compromise placental circulation and negatively impact the fetus's well-being. In my experience, unnecessary delays caused by incompetent obstetricians are a significant factor in harm to the baby's brain. Unfortunately, these delays are often overlooked or attributed to other factors.

Other complications associated with cesarean sections are similar to those found in any abdominal or pelvic surgery. Common issues include injuries to the bladder, rectum, and ureters. Additional complications may involve excessive bleeding, bowel perforation, and trauma to the fetal head. Later complications can arise, such as wound infections, ileus (a condition affecting the motility of intestines), and the formation of fistulas.

Despite advances in anesthesia techniques and improved obstetrical training, infant and maternal mortality rates remain high in the United States, particularly for Black Americans (see Figures 7-2 and 7-3).

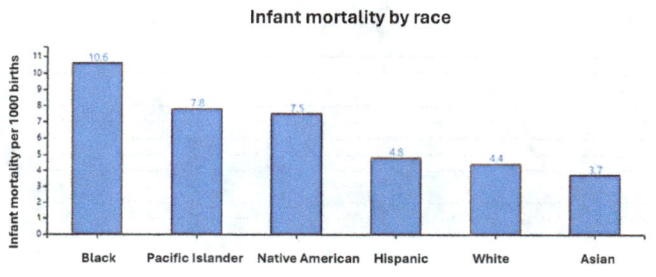

Figure 7-3. Infant mortality by race in the US (2022).

Chapter 8

HOLISTIC METHODS OF PAIN RELIEF

In this chapter, we will explore various holistic pain relief options. Many cultures around the world, unaffected by Western influence, have developed natural coping mechanisms for managing labor pain. Holistic methods refer to non-mainstream pain relief techniques that are not commonly utilized in Western medicine. The term "holistic" encompasses approaches that consider the individual as a whole—mentally and physically—helping them withstand the challenges of labor. More accurately, these interventions can be defined as integrative medicine approaches to pain relief.

The alternative and complementary techniques discussed here should ideally be practiced alongside providers trained in Western medicine. Western medicine and holistic options are not mutually exclusive; mothers can and should integrate elements from both approaches. Attempting holistic methods without the safety net of modern obstetrical care would be unwise.

The holistic approach to labor is a continuum that begins with conception and extends beyond labor into the postpartum period. In addition to pain relief strategies during labor, this approach encompasses education, proper nutrition, physical fitness, mental resilience, and achieving spiritual harmony with the processes of life and birth.

For clarity, we will categorize holistic pain relief modalities into physical, mental, nutritional, and herbal methods, as illustrated in Figure 8-1. We will discuss these methods in the order of interventions applicable during pregnancy and those suitable for labor.

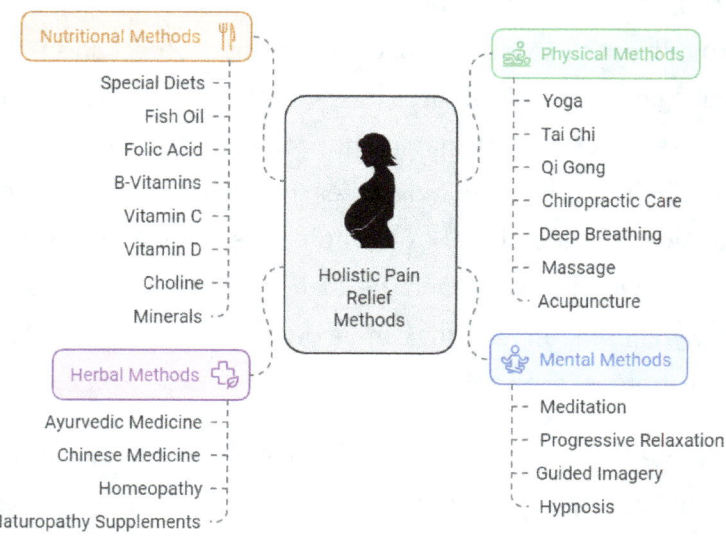

Figure 8-1. Holistic approaches to pain relief during pregnancy and labor.

Physical Activity

The importance of physical fitness during labor and delivery cannot be overemphasized. Women with the stamina, endurance, strength, and flexibility often breeze through labor and delivery. They suffer fewer complications and report positive experiences.

Physically deconditioned women suffer from exhaustion and protracted labor, have difficulty pushing, and experience shortness of breath during the later phases of stage one and stage two. There are also observational studies that suggest physically deconditioned women suffer more frequent protracted labor and C-sections.

Therefore, it is advisable for women already practicing fitness arts such as yoga, tai chi, or qi gong to continue these exercises during pregnancy. These techniques concentrate on joint flexibility, balance, and breathing; all three will help immensely during labor. You should also avoid high-impact exercises, contact sports, and physical activities in low-oxygen partial pressure environments such as high altitudes.

Pregnant women should perform at least 30 minutes of aerobic activity every day. Care must be taken to stay within one's comfort zone and not push beyond the threshold of pain. If you have diabetes, hypertension, anemia, heart disease, placenta previa, twin pregnancy, or preeclampsia, please consult your prenatal care provider to determine what level of exercise is appropriate.

Nutritional Intake During Pregnancy

A pregnant woman needs to eat a balanced diet of carbohydrates, proteins, fat, vitamins, and minerals. The total caloric intake should be 2,400 calories per day during the first trimester, increasing by 340 calories during the second and third trimesters. During the second and third trimesters, the weight gain should be no more than one pound a week. Most women gain 24 to 36 pounds during pregnancy. In women with diabetes and preeclampsia, the weight gain may be far more than this range.

World Health Organization data shows that preterm birth, low birth weight, and stillbirth are significantly greater in women who suffer protein-calorie malnutrition during pregnancy. It is recommended that pregnant women consume 1.1 grams per kilogram of body weight per day of protein during the second and third trimesters.

Fat intake is an essential part of a balanced diet during pregnancy; however, fat should constitute no more than 25 to 35 percent of the total caloric intake per day.

The need for an adequate intake of vitamins and minerals cannot be overemphasized. Several ailments manifest in the infant and the mother when the levels of specific micronutrients are inadequate in the diet. For example, adequate iron intake can eliminate anemia in the mother and low birth weight in the infant. Spina bifida in infants can be prevented by proper supplementation with folic acid in the diet.

Some common diseases caused by deficiency of vitamins and minerals are summarized in Table 8-1 [41] and Table 8-2 [42]. (*RDAs shown in the tables have been modified from Dietary Guidelines for Americans 2020 to 2025.)

VITAMIN	DAILY DOSE*	DEFICIENCY IN MOTHER	DEFICIENCY IN INFANT
Vitamin A	770 mcg	Anemia Night blindness Preeclampsia Eclampsia	Heart defects Orofacial defects Impaired lung function
Vitamin C	85 mg	Premature rupture of membrane Abdominal pain Preeclampsia Urinary tract infection	Wheeze Impaired lung function Low birth weight Orofacial cleft
Vitamin D	600 IU	Increase cesarean section Preeclampsia Hypertension Infections Secondary hyperparathyroidism	Autism Preterm birth Asthma Miscarriage Language difficulties Impaired psychomotor skills
Vitamin E	15 mg	Premature rupture of membrane Eclampsia Hyperglycemia Insulin resistance	Heart defects Orofacial defects Preterm birth Placental abruption Wheeze
Vitamin K	90 mcg	Gestational diabetes Postpartum depression	Intracranial hemorrhage Excessive bleeding
Vitamin B1 (Thiamine)	1.4 mg	Glucose intolerance	Anencephaly Low birth weight Learning disabilities
Vitamin B2 (Riboflavin)	1.4 mg	Anemia Night blindness Hypertension Preeclampsia	Low birth weight Birth defects Heart defects
Vitamin B3 (Niacin)	18 mg	Preeclampsia Gestational hypertension	Spina bifida Heart defects Low birth weight

Table 8-1. Essential vitamins for healthy pregnancy.

MINERAL	DAILY DOSE*	DEFICIENCY IN MOTHER	DEFICIENCY IN INFANT
Iron	27 mg	Anemia	Anemia Anencephaly Autism Orofacial cleft Low birth weight
Copper	1 mg	Anxiety Blighted ovum Depression Miscarriage	Anencephaly CNS malformations
Magnesium	360 mg	Edema Gestational hypertension Preeclampsia Leg cramps	Low Apgar score Low birth weight Cerebral palsy Preterm birth Orofacial cleft
Selenium	70 mcg	Edema Gestational hypertension Preeclampsia Hypothyroidism Miscarriage Gestational diabetes Infections	Neural tube defects Low birth weight Congenital Diaphragmatic hernia Intellectual disability
Chromium	30 mcg	Gestational diabetes Postpartum depression	
Calcium	1,000 mg	Gestational hypertension Preeclampsia Maternal death	Autism Preterm birth Rickets Dental cavities Low birth weight
Iodine	220 mcg	Hypothyroidism Preeclampsia	Hypothyroidism ADD ADHD Autism Intellectual disability Infant mortality
Zinc	11 mg	Preeclampsia Gestational hypertension	Preterm birth Low Apgar scores Low birth weight Impetigo Asthma Wheeze
Manganese	2 mg		Preterm birth Low birth weight Intellectual disability

Table 8-2. Essential minerals for healthy pregnancy.

However, a detailed discussion of your specific nutritional deficiencies and their adverse impacts on your pregnancy is beyond

the scope of this text. Mothers interested in more information should visit the US Department of Health and Human Services, Office of Disease Prevention and Health Promotion website (https://odphp.health.gov/) and have a detailed discussion with their healthcare providers.

Yoga During Pregnancy

Yoga is the ancient Indian art of practicing physical postures, relaxation, and controlled breathing to achieve optimal health and mind-body-spirit harmony. A systematic analysis of published clinical trials showed that yoga practiced during the prenatal period reduced anxiety, stress, and duration of labor while it increased the odds of vaginal childbirth and tolerance to pain [43].

The magic of yoga lies in its simplicity in preparing you for stress-free childbirth. Yoga is complementary and can be effectively used with any other conventional interventions if the parturient desires. Yoga studios and gyms offer prenatal yoga classes in many cities and towns. Instructor-led courses are motivating and enjoyable.

However, some basic precautions must be taken. If you feel pain from a posture, do not proceed; stop and reassess. If it happens again, then that posture should be avoided. Do not over-stretch your limbs or spine. You should have a partner, friend, or instructor observing and helping you if you need assistance.

During the second and third trimesters, avoid postures that press on the abdomen, as this could cause injury to the fetus or precipitate labor. During the third trimester, do not perform any posture that requires lying flat on your back. In doing so, the gravid uterus compresses the inferior vena cava and, to some degree, the abdominal aorta against the lumbar vertebrae. This compression diminishes the amount of venous blood returning to the heart and reduces the cardiac output, causing low blood pressure and a shock-like state. About 15 to 20 percent of women complain of feeling nauseous and lightheaded while in this position. This condition is called ***aortocaval compression syndrome***. Left uncorrected for any length of time, it can compromise the perfusion of the placenta and lead to oxygen and nutrient deprivation of the fetus. The remedy is to turn and lie on your left side. You can also sit up or stand. These measures unload the pressure on the vena cava and the aorta, quickly restoring normal blood pressure.

Listing all the postures (called *asanas*) that can be safely practiced during pregnancy is beyond the scope of this book; anyone interested in learning more can easily find resources on the internet. However, a few seminal postures known to be beneficial during various stages of pregnancy are discussed on the following pages. The postures shown are basic and targeted for beginners in yoga.

During the first trimester, concentrate on strengthening and improving the stability of your pelvis, spine, and lower limb muscles and joints. The postures should enhance spinal stability, balance, and flexibility. Some instructors recommend the lotus pose, the warrior pose, and the downward-facing dog pose.

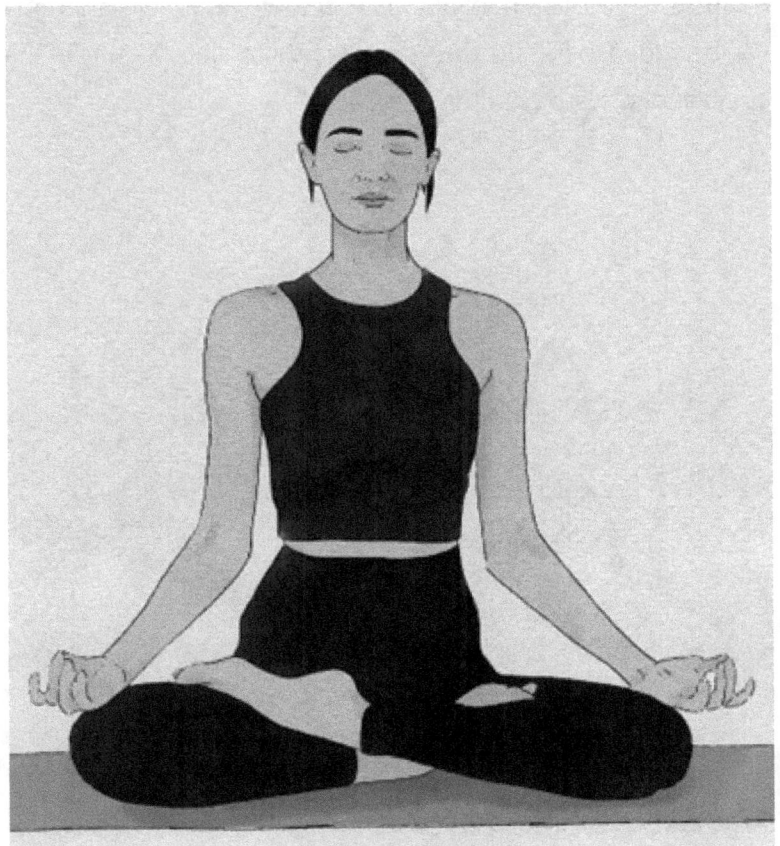

Figure 8-2. Lotus pose.

To achieve the lotus pose (*padmasana*) as shown in Figure 8-2, sit cross-legged on the mat. Pull the abdomen in and keep the spine erect so the lower back, shoulders, and the back of the head are straight and perpendicular to the floor. The shoulders are relaxed, and the hands rest on the knees, with palms facing upward. The chin is parallel to the ground, and the eyes are half closed, gazing downward. Calm your mind and concentrate on slow, deep breathing. This posture can be maintained for several minutes. If you're already familiar with yoga, other variations can be added to this posture, such as side-to-side twisting of the spine and forward bending at the waist.

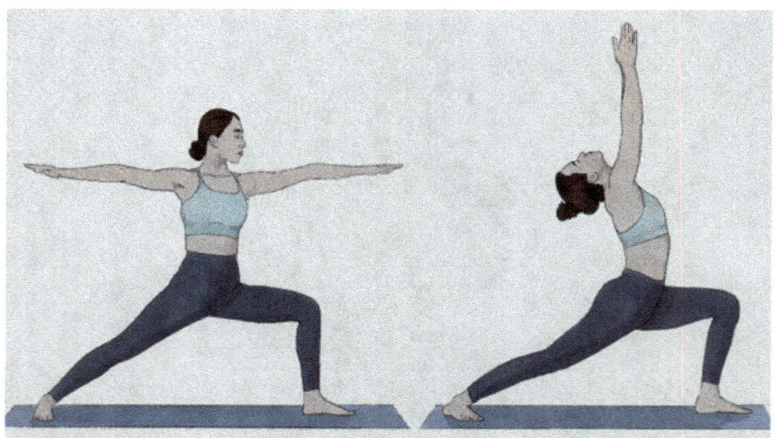

Figure 8-3. Warrior pose.

To achieve the warrior pose (*virabhadrasana*) as shown in Figure 8-3, stand with your feet apart, at least two to three times the width of your shoulders. Then, raise your arms parallel to the ground, palms facing down. Slowly turn one foot 90 degrees to the side and bend your knee so the thigh is parallel to the ground. Turn your head to the same side and keep your gaze afar. Hold this posture for a few minutes then gradually turn your shoulders and chest to the same side, raise your arms, clasp your hands, and reach high toward the ceiling. You should feel the stretch from your toes to the fingers. Hold this posture for a few minutes and repeat the process on the other side.

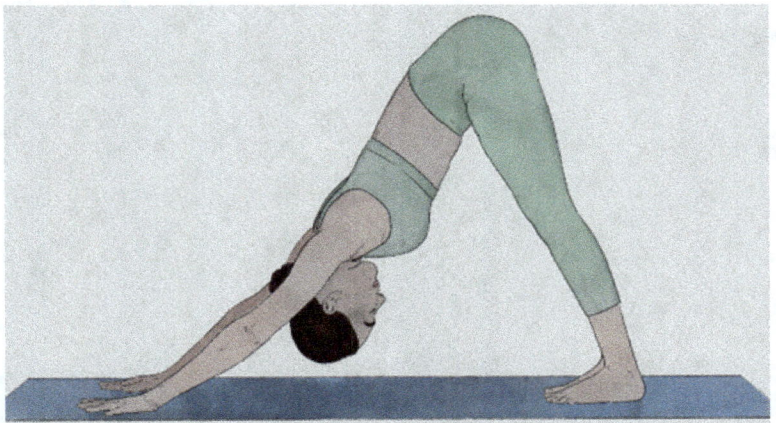

Figure 8-4. Downward-facing dog.

To achieve the downward-facing dog pose (*adho mukha svanasana*) as shown in Figure 8-4, begin on all fours, with hands and feet firmly planted on the mat. The feet must be separated at least shoulder length apart, and the knees bent. Then, slowly lift your hips upward, straightening your knees and elbows until you feel the stretch in your legs, hamstrings, back, and arms. You may have to move your back and legs apart if the stretch is uncomfortable or challenging to perform. Gaze toward your feet and breathe slowly and deeply. In this posture, your head will be lower than your heart, and you'll feel your head and neck engorged with blood. Hold this posture for a few minutes, then buckle your knees and rise from this posture carefully and slowly.

During the second trimester, work on various postures and proper breathing. The goal is to learn deep breathing and proper pushing techniques. Some generally recommended postures include the diamond pose, the cobbler pose, and the bridge pose.

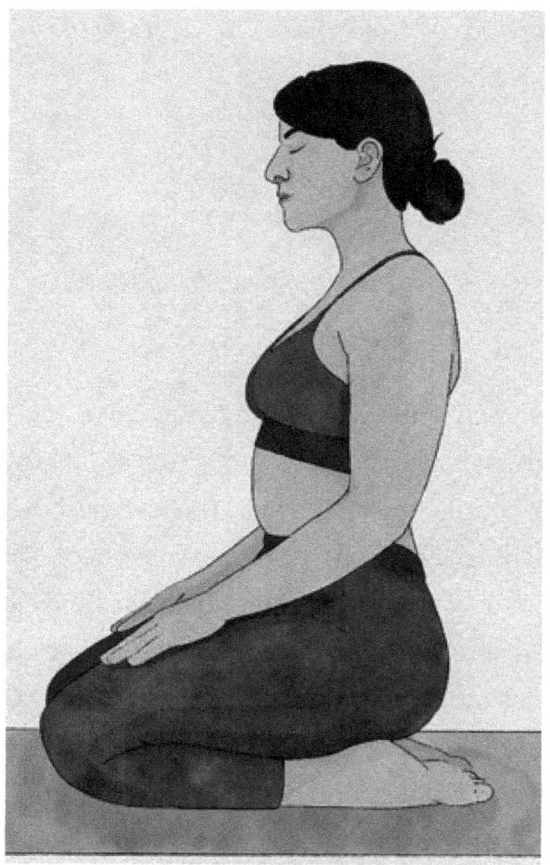

Figure 8-5. Diamond pose.

The diamond pose (*vajrasana*) as shown in Figure 8-5, improves flexibility in your knees, hips, and ankles. You begin by kneeling with your feet extended, the great toes slightly touching, and the heels rotated outward. Then, gently lower your buttocks to rest on your heels. Bring your spine erect, chin up, and gaze forward. Straighten your elbows and rest your hands over your knees. Allow your abdomen to move freely with your respirations. Hold this posture for five to seven minutes.

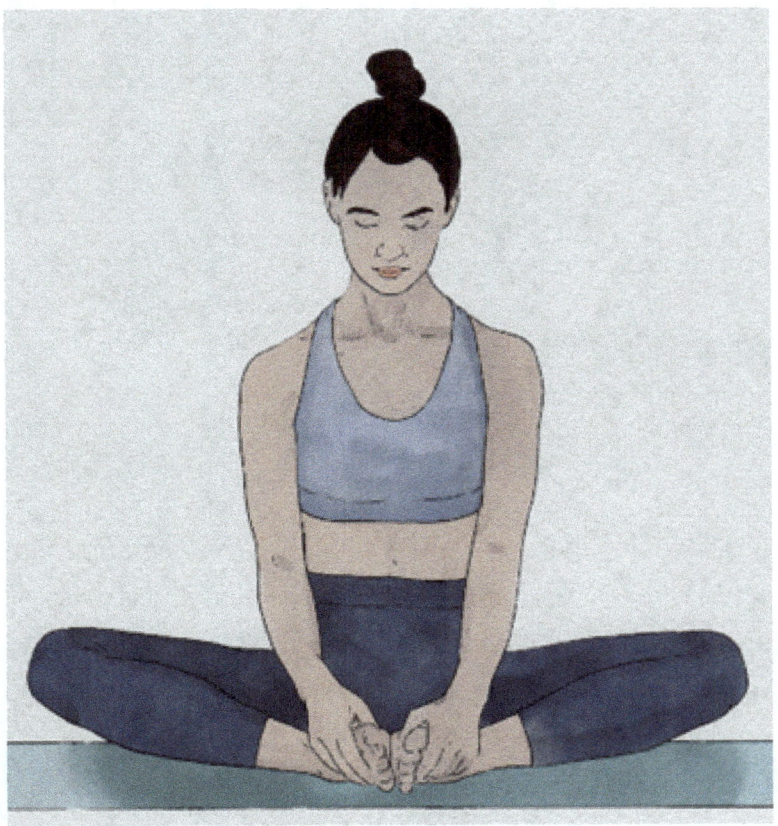

Figure 8-6. Cobbler's pose.

As shown in Figure 8-6, the cobbler's pose (*baddha konasana*) helps stretch your hip joints, pelvic ring, and knees and improves your posture and balance. You begin by sitting on the mat with your legs stretched out. Then, you should align your feet, soles touching each other, and pull them slowly toward your groin. Allow your knees to bend and fall toward the mat. Straighten both elbows and grab your feet's outer margins. Keep your spine erect and breathe slowly, relaxing your hips and pelvic muscles. Maintain the posture for several minutes.

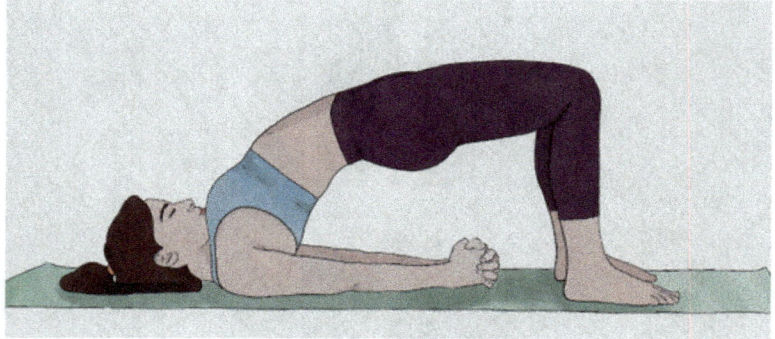

Figure 8-7. Bridge pose.

As shown in Figure 8-7, the bridge pose (*setu bandhasana*) works with the core muscles of your abdomen, gluteal muscles, and hamstrings. It helps stabilize the pelvis, adds flexibility to the lumbar and thoracic spine, and improves circulation to the head and neck. For this pose, first lie flat on the mat, flex your hips and knees, and bring your feet toward your hip joints. Lay your arms on your side and push down with your arms while slowly straightening your hips and raising the pelvis toward the ceiling. Your feet must remain flat on the mat, with knees flexed and hips extended. Breathe slowly and keep the posture for two to three minutes. Stop if you feel lightheaded or like your heart is racing. Lie on your left side or sit up.

During the third trimester, concentrate on relaxing and stretching your hip joints, knees, and lower back muscles and ligaments. The goal is to prepare the pelvic outlet for the baby's transit. Some of the recommended postures are the garland pose, the cat and cow pose, and the goddess pose.

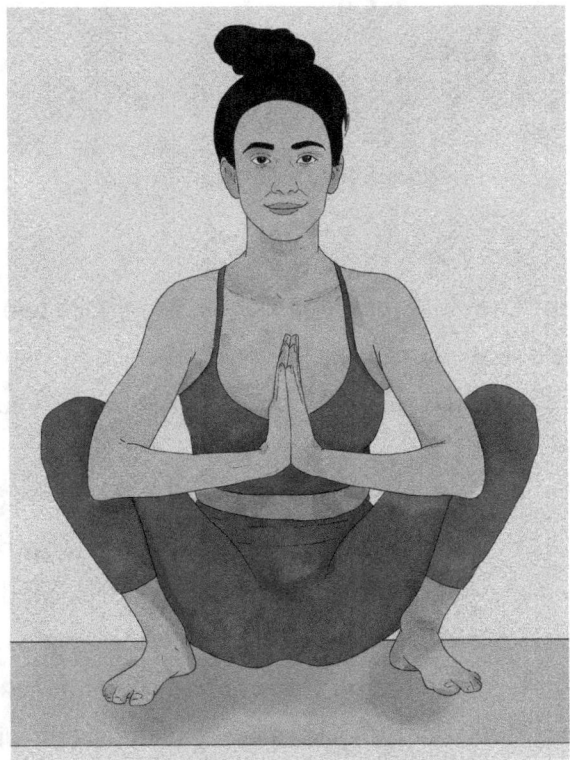

Figure 8-8. Garland Pose.

To achieve the garland pose (*malasana*) as shown in Figure 8-8, gently squat with your feet slightly wider than your pelvis and turned at 45 degrees. Clasp your hands in front of the sternum. Keep your spine erect. Concentrate on slow, deep breathing and relaxing your hips and pelvic musculature. Maintain the pose for a few minutes, then relax and stand up. Repeat this cycle about 10 times.

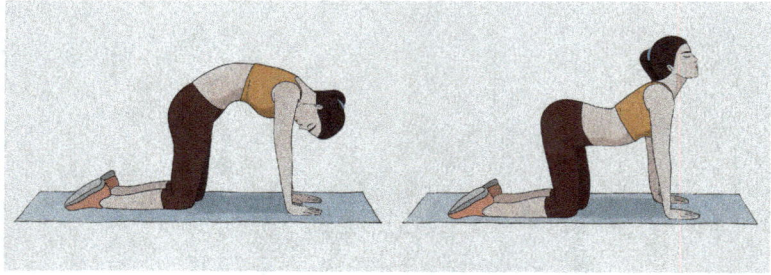

Figure 8-9. Cat and cow pose.

The cat and cow pose (*marjariasana-bitilisana*) are two exercises done sequentially, causing flexion and extension of the entire spine, as shown in Figure 8-9. Start the exercises on your hands and knees. Gently arch your spine toward the ceiling and lower your head to place your chin on your sternum. Pull your hips and pelvis to create an arch (some call it the rainbow posture). Breathe slowly and hold the posture for several seconds. Then, slowly relax your lower back and arch the spine toward the floor. Raise your head and extend your cervical spine to look toward the ceiling. Push your hips and pelvis out and up, allowing your abdomen and uterus to hang freely due to gravity. Hold the posture for a few minutes, then relax. Repeat this flexion and extension of the spine about 10 times.

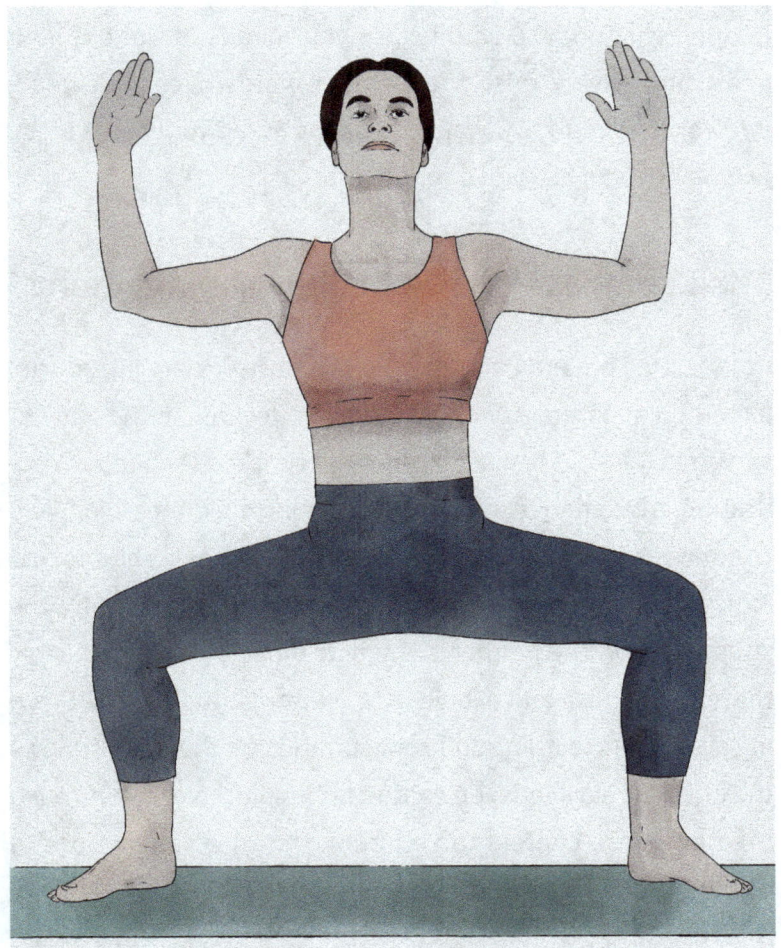

Figure 8-10. Goddess pose.

To achieve the goddess pose (*utkata konasana*) as shown in Figure 8-10, stand with your feet apart and your toes turned outward and stretched out. Then, slowly bend your knees to a half squat. Next, bend your elbows and wrists to half flexion. Breathe slowly, keep this posture for a few minutes, and then rise. Repeat this 10 times.

In one variation, you could clasp your hands in front of your chest and slowly raise the clasped hands over your head, stretching your arms toward the ceiling. Keep your spine erect, and do not lean forward or backward.

The Lamaze Method of Labor Management

In 1951, Dr. Fernand Lamaze, a French obstetrician, introduced a method of natural childbirth based on techniques he had observed in Russia. The Lamaze method consists of childbirth education, relaxation techniques, deep controlled breathing, and continuous emotional support from the partner. The process aims to build confidence and provide coping strategies for the stress of labor. The mother is taught to inhale slowly and deeply through the nose and exhale slowly through the mouth. Slowing down the breathing and concentrating on the breath allows the body to relax between contractions completely. Controlled breathing also centers the mind on the singular purpose of birthing and blocks out extraneous distractions.

Many women find the Lamaze techniques useful in other stressful situations (Figure 8-11), such as controlling their emotions and overcoming pain. Lamaze techniques are fully compatible with other forms of pain management, including epidurals. All pregnant women, whether they are planning on a natural birth or not, should undergo some form of Lamaze training, either in person or through online classes.

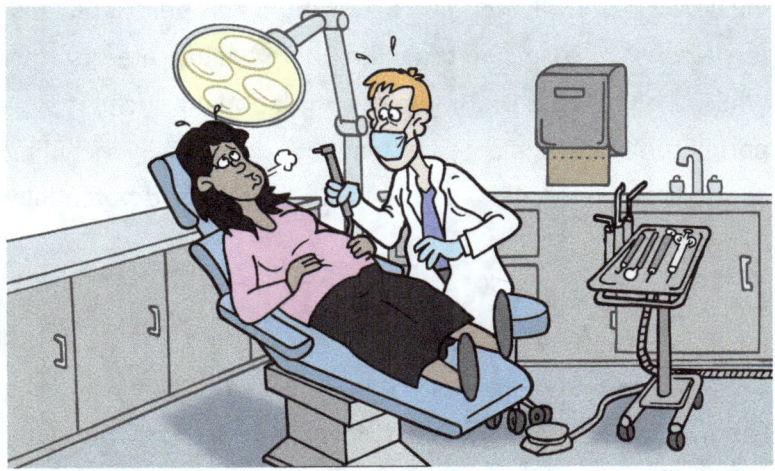

Figure 8-11. "Hold on!" cried Ms. Wedel, "let me do my Lamaze breathing before you drill!"

The Bradley Method of Labor Management

In 1965, Dr. Robert Bradley, an American obstetrician, proposed going back to natural childbirth without the use of surgery, medications, or any other allopathic (or more conventional) interventions. He advocated for babies to be born without the adverse effects of drugs and trauma from surgical interventions. His philosophy emphasizes deep breathing and concentration on expelling the fetus with each contraction in an environment without distractions. Education, preparation, and the participation of a loving partner were cornerstones of the Bradley method. It was also crucial for the mother to remain physically and mentally healthy to avoid complications during labor and remain strong to withstand the rigors of birthing. The Bradley method opposes any form of conventional intervention, including intravenous infusions and medication. This philosophy fosters a sense of suspicion toward modern health-care systems. While I believe that Dr. Bradley's foundational principles support natural birth and are commendable, deliberately excluding all medical interventions may be unnecessary and potentially dangerous.

Water Birth

Laboring and birthing in water have been practiced in many parts of Asia, Russia, and France. The warmth and buoyancy of the water help relax the pelvic muscles and provide a modest amount of pain relief and comfort. Several studies show a shorter duration of labor and a reduction in the number of cesarean sections with water tubs. Most women report positive experiences with water laboring and request water tubs for subsequent labor. Many modern hospitals have large bathing tubs, similar to Jacuzzi tubs, right in the birthing room. The mother is encouraged to stay in the water for phase one of labor. Once the cervix is fully dilated and the baby's head is present at the perineum, the mother is transferred to her bed and out of the water for the delivery.

Birthing can happen in the water if your obstetrician or midwife is trained and experienced in delivering babies in water. However, the advantage of stepping away from the tub water for the delivery is that it avoids accidental aspiration of the tub water by the baby when she or he attempts to breathe. Unless the obstetrician or the midwife is fast enough to raise the baby's head out of the water, small amounts of water will enter the baby's mouth. The baby must then be held upside down, and the mouth and pharynx suctioned clear. The aspiration of contaminated tub water into the lungs could lead to severe lung infection in the newborn baby.

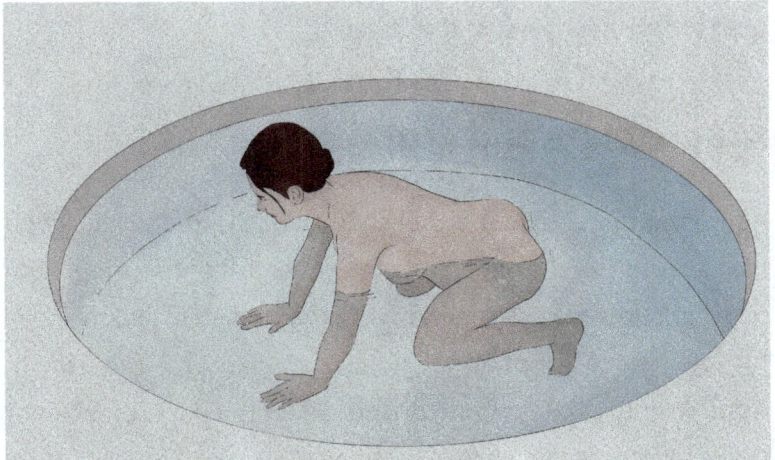

Figure 8-12. Parturient on hands and knees in a "doggy position" inside the water tub.

Additionally, it is vitally important that sufficient help is available to assist the mother in getting in and out of the water tub. Accidental slips and falls could be catastrophic for the mother and the child. There must be a minimum of two assistants holding the mother on either side as she gets in and out of the tub. The water must be clean and warm. No perfumes, soaps, or other chemicals should be added to the water. There must be an easily accessible large drain, should it become necessary to deliver in the tub.

Most mothers find resting on their knees and hands, with water up to their neck, allowing the abdomen to hang freely in the water, to be the most comfortable position (Figure 8-12). Some prefer to sit at the edge of the tub. It's important to allow the mother to choose the most comfortable position. It's best to wait to start any intravenous lines or apply monitoring leads until the mother is out of the water.

Acupuncture and Acupressure

A systematic review of the published medical literature suggests that acupuncture is only marginally effective in reducing labor pain [44]. However, satisfaction with the pain relief and the need for lower doses of pharmacological agents were reported in Asian women. Acupuncture did not affect the duration of labor or the incidence of cesarean section.

According to traditional Chinese medicine, the life force (qi) flows along certain meridians discernible on the body surface. Disease or pain manifests when this normal flow is interrupted, causing an imbalance of yin and yang, the opposing forces within the body that, under normal circumstances, exist in a dynamic equilibrium. When qi is stagnant or misdirected, the yin-yang equilibrium is upset, resulting in disease or pain. Needling (acupuncture) or massaging (acupressure) specific points along the meridian resets the flow of qi, resulting in the abatement of pain and the disease process.

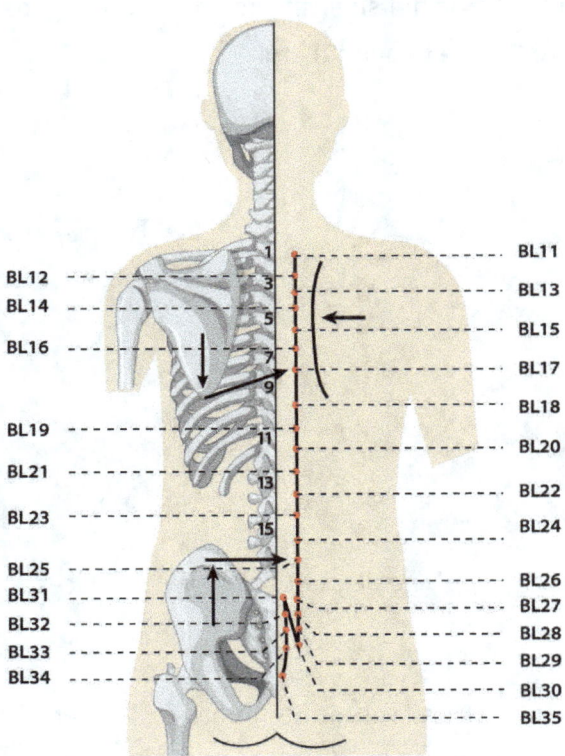

Figure 8-13. Acupuncture points in the back.

Acupuncture: This process involves placing 10 to 20 fine needles into the skin along the meridians in the lower back. There are several points along the paravertebral meridian (Figure 8-13), ranging from T10 to L3 and the para-sacral gluteal dimples, that are chosen for stimulation [45]. The needles are gently moved or twirled to stimulate the nerve endings in the skin.

Heat or mild electrical current might be applied to stimulate the nerves better. The needles are left in place for 20 to 30 minutes and removed. The process can be repeated several times until the very late phase of stage one labor. The parturient must be on her side, sitting up or standing, to achieve the best response to acupuncture.

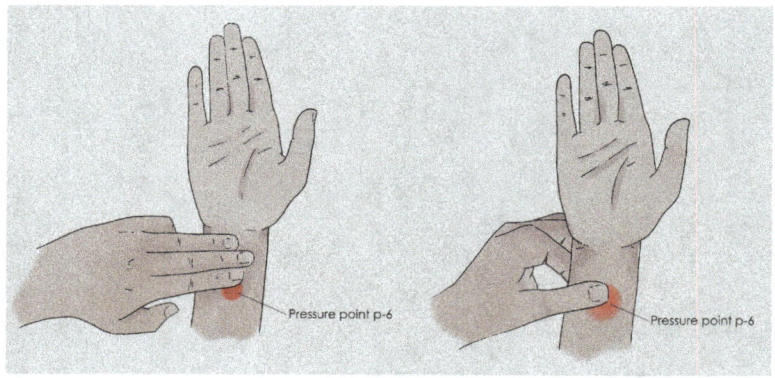

Figure 8-14. Applying pressure to point P-6 reduces nausea.

Acupressure: This technique involves the partner or the healthcare provider gently rubbing the lower back of the parturient with their hands. Gradually, firm pressure must be applied to the region just lateral to the L2 vertebrae. The thumb or the knuckles of two fingers may apply pressure of about 10 to 20 pounds for 20 to 30 seconds. Then, the hands slowly move down toward the sacrum, and pressure is applied to the dimple on either side of the S2 vertebrae. Acupressure is best performed between contractions until the fetal head shows in the perineum.

Other helpful acupressure points are located at P-6 (as seen in Figure 8-14) and L14 (as seen in Figure 8-15). Pressure applied with the thumb in a vertical pinching fashion often reduces or terminates the feeling of nausea. Pressure at L14 may also aid in reducing the intensity of labor pain.

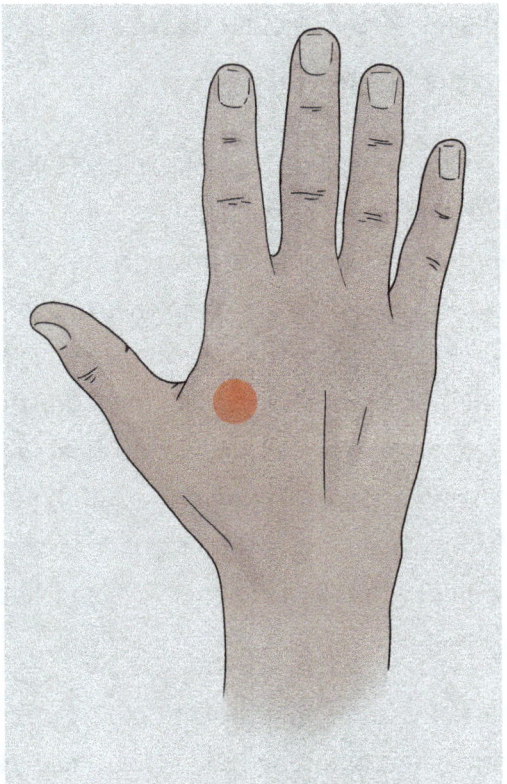

*Figure 8-15. Pressure applied to point L14
(He Gu) can reduce labor pain.*

There are few to no side effects of acupuncture or acupressure. Rarely, if the needles are not sterilized properly, puncturing the skin can lead to local or systemic infection. Minor bleeding and hematoma formation can occur in women who are on anticoagulants. More often, the parturients complain of sharp pain at the site of needle insertion, nausea, or lightheadedness. These symptoms resolve upon removal or repositioning of the needles.

Transcutaneous Electrical Nerve Stimulation (TENS)

Transcutaneous electrical nerve stimulation (TENS) is based on the principle that, when a less painful stimulus is applied to a nerve, more painful stimuli are prevented from entering the spinal cord nerve cells. This is often referred to as the gate control theory of pain perception. TENS works by applying less painful stimuli in the form of electrical stimulation through electrodes applied to the same skin innervation areas (dermatomes) of the spinal nerves supplying deeper painful organs (Figure 8-16). To block the pain sensations emanating from the uterus, the dermatomes L2 to T10 will need to be stimulated with electrical impulses.

TENS units are modestly effective in the early stage one of labor. The stimulation must be strong enough to be mildly uncomfortable and could be left on between contractions. One could keep the stimulation on for 30 minutes and off for 30 minutes and repeat the cycle several times. Studies show that continuous stimulation through TENS electrodes may increase endorphins in the spinal cord, which are natural painkillers.

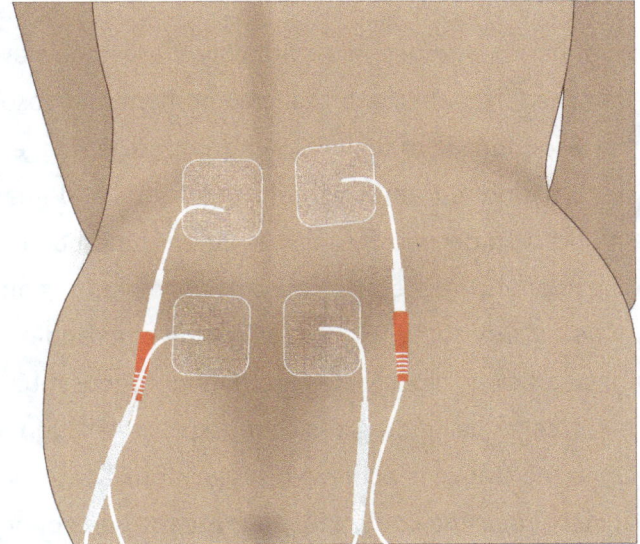

Figure 8-16. Transcutaneous electrical nerve stimulation (TENS) leads are applied to the lower back.

In my experience, most women want the device turned off as the labor progresses and the cervix nears full dilatation. They report the stimulations to be more annoying than helpful at this stage. This may be a natural physiological response as the body quickly develops resistance to any beneficial effects of electrical stimulation due to neuronal fatigue or tachyphylaxis.

The bottom line is that TENS can be beneficial in the early stages of labor when used for a few hours, but don't expect significant pain relief from these devices. They pose little or no harm to the mother or the baby.

Hypnotherapy

Hypnosis is a trance-like state where a person's awareness is detached from their external environment and absorbed by inner experiences of feelings, emotions, and imagery [46]. Under a hypnotic trance, verbal suggestions and imagery direct the brain to desired feelings, emotions, and bodily responses. The hypnotic trance is achieved by concentrating on a monotonous sensory stimulus, such as staring at a candle flame, looking at a ticking clock, listening to monotonous music, chanting mantras, or using progressive muscular relaxation techniques. Once the trance is achieved, suggestions are given to reduce anxiety, relax the body, and minimize the perceptions of pain.

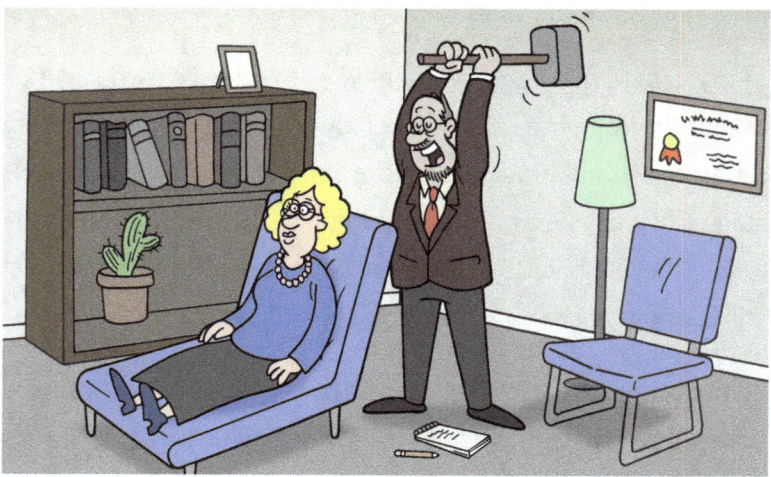

Figure 8-17. "Relax, Ms. Arendt, we will now transition from your subconscious to your unconscious!"

In institutions that offer hypnotherapy, expecting mothers are taught self-hypnosis in four to six sessions, each lasting about 90 minutes during the third trimester. During these sessions, the women are taught how to relax through hypnosis and provided with imagery of labor and delivery. Suggestions are made regarding how labor pain should be processed and experienced as natural and not harmful. Mentally rehearsing the labor and delivery takes away from the anxiety related to the unknown and prepares women for the actual day of labor and delivery. The women's partners are instructed to assist with relaxation, deep breathing, and pushing during delivery.

On the day of delivery, the women self-induce a hypnotic trance with the onset of regular contractions. Most prefer to listen to audio recordings from prior sessions to transition into the trance state effortlessly. Once in a hypnotic trance, auto-suggestions on the benefits of the contractions and the tolerability of the pain, coupled with the imagery of the baby, help mask the pain of the contractions. Some hospitals allow the hypnotherapist to be at the parturient's bedside, facilitate the induction of hypnotic trance, and provide positive suggestions for relaxation and pain control. The woman's partner may also assume the role of the hypnotherapist.

Hypnotherapy is said to utilize the power of suggestion to control the pain, breathe deeply, relax, and achieve a tranquil state conducive to natural childbirth. Systematic analyses of published clinical trials show a meager reduction in the use of pain medications with hypnosis. Many women and healthcare providers find it difficult to accept that controlling the subconscious mind can reduce physical pain (Figure 8-17). Studies show no demonstrable differences between women in the hypnosis group and those in the control groups for satisfaction with pain relief, sense of coping with labor, the need for a rescue epidural, or spontaneous vaginal birth [47]. At the present time, more rigorous clinical studies are needed to determine the merits of hypnotherapy.

In my opinion, hypnotherapy can serve as a powerful adjunct to other modalities of pain management. However, used as the sole method of pain control, it might not be sufficient except in 10 to 15 percent of the most highly motivated and well-informed parturients.

Massage

As a detailed discussion on the role of massage in pregnancy and labor is beyond the scope of this book, we will cover the basics here. There are several schools of massage. Massage therapists are constantly innovating new techniques and instruments (Figure 8-18). During pregnancy, the Swedish style of massage is often considered the best option. It involves the following:

- **Effleurage**: long, smooth, firm, gliding strokes over the skin to relax the soft tissue

- **Petrissage**: the squeezing, pinching, rolling, or kneading of the muscles

- **Friction**: deep, concentric movements with firm pressure that cause layers of tissue to rub against each other, increasing the circulation of blood and lymphatic fluid

- **Tapotement**: short, alternating taps performed with cupped hands, fingertips, or the edge of the hands to improve circulation and stimulate the nerve endings in muscles

If you have markers for a high-risk pregnancy, such as preeclampsia, twins, or placenta previa, then massages around the abdomen and pelvis should generally be avoided. In otherwise healthy mothers, massages performed once or twice a week for 20 to 30 minutes have been shown to reduce anxiety, relax the muscles, provide restorative sleep, and increase the sense of well-being. It reduces the stress hormones and increases the calming hormones such as serotonin, dopamine, and endorphins.

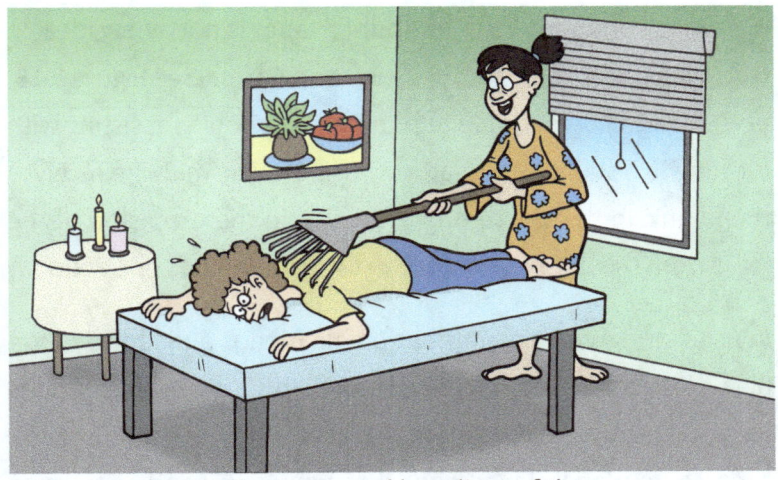

Figure 8-18. Sandra reassured her client of the new massage technique called "rakey, rakey!"

More importantly, massages provided by a loving partner improve the bonding between partners and the baby in the womb. Psychologically, they show commitment from both the mother and the father toward the family's well-being and set the entire pregnancy and labor on the path to being a joint family effort.

Massaging the lower back, shoulders, and neck during labor reduces anxiety, relaxes the pelvic musculature, and improves breathing. Massages are best performed between contractions in the first stage of labor. During the active second stage, when the fetal head is at the vaginal outlet, it's best to hold off on massages and concentrate on straining and pushing. A gentle massage may be continued after the birth of the baby and the delivery of the placenta. This will enhance the sense of achievement, relaxation, and euphoria.

Continuous Support

Receiving continuous support during labor is not a new idea. In fact, it's as old as human civilizations on Earth. (See Figure 8-19, in which a 2,000-year-old sculpture depicts doulas assisting with birthing in a standing, squatting position. The midwife receives the infant. In this posture, gravity aids in the expulsion of the fetus from the uterus without the need for forceps or traction.)

In Asian and African countries, female friends and family members are continuously present during labor and birth, supporting and encouraging the mother. It comes naturally in most cultures to help one's loved ones through painful and distressing situations. They hold the mother's hands, help them settle in a comfortable posture, engage in comforting talk, breathe with the mother, encourage her to push with the contractions, and help visualize the joy of birthing. They unequivocally declare they will remain with the parturient every step of the way until the baby is born. Their affirmation of continuous presence provides the laboring mother with an abundance of safety, security, and comfort.

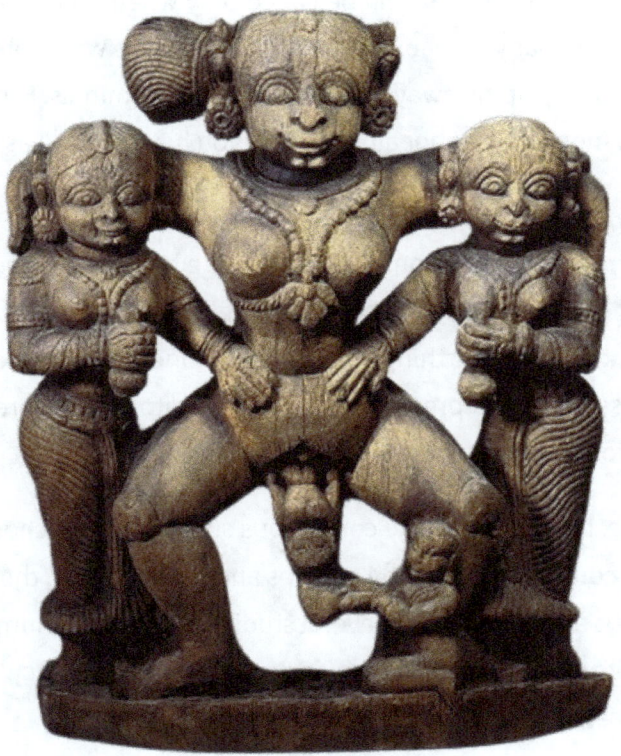

Figure 8-19. A stone carving from the 2,000-year-old Pungampadi Shiva Temple in Tamil Nadu, India.

These support women are the forerunners of the doulas we see making a resurgence in the United States today, which are being reintroduced out of necessity. It's a tragedy that, in modern labor and delivery suites, some women labor alone or with just a spouse sitting there watching TV.

Don't expect the nurses or the obstetrician to stay with you while enduring labor pains. The nurse may come in to start your IV, put on the monitors, and then promptly leave your bedside. The anesthesiologist will place the epidural, write orders, and walk away. The obstetrician will be called only when there's a problem or the baby is ready for delivery. Everyone will pretend to be too busy, typing away on their computer terminals. Expect to spend most of the labor alone unless you have a doula assisting you.

In my opinion, a woman walking into the hospital alone to deliver her baby is one of the most tragic sights to behold. For them, the whole birthing experience is lonely, miserable, sad, distressing, and depressing. They also tend to suffer more complications and unnecessary cesarean sections.

Doulas, however, provide continuous support. If one chooses a doula compatible with one's values and expectations, the experience is almost magical. Several studies have shown numerous benefits to having a doula provide care during pregnancy, labor, and postpartum. These benefits include the following:

- Increased spontaneous vaginal births

- Shorter duration of labor

- Decrease in cesarean sections

- Decrease in instrumented vaginal delivery

- Decreased use of opioid analgesics

- Decreased need for epidural analgesia

- Improved Apgar scores in the infant

- Increased breastfeeding rates

- Enhanced mother-infant bonding

- Lowered incidence of postpartum depression [48]

In my experience, an overwhelming majority of women express satisfaction and joy with the contributions of the doula to their birthing experience. Doulas are particularly effective in reducing anxiety and providing comfort during instrumental delivery or C-section, where your spouse might not know how to be supportive (Figure 8-20). Except for a few interpersonal conflicts that might arise between the doulas and the medical staff, there are no real downsides to doulas providing continuous support.

Doulas are so effective in improving outcomes for the mother and the baby that the March of Dimes Foundation has developed a position statement urging increased access to doulas, insurance coverage for doula services, and improved training and certification of doulas. Doulas of North America, a nonprofit foundation created in 1992, currently provides training and certification for doulas. Their vision is "a doula for every person who wants one." Their standards of practice and code of ethics are listed on their website (www.dona.org).

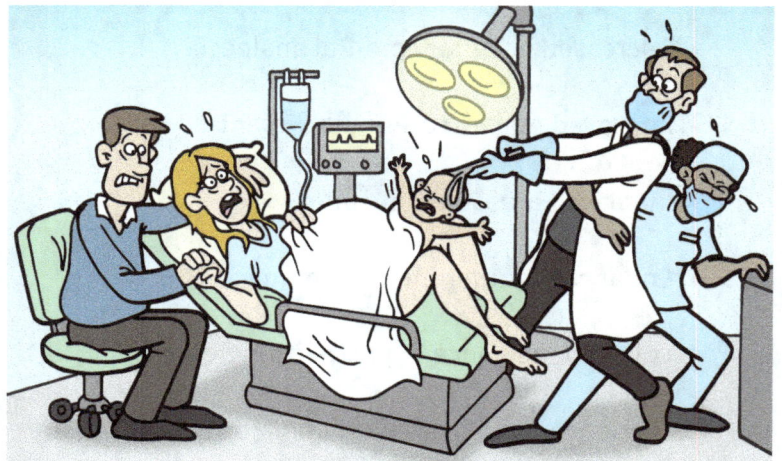

Figure 8-20. Dr. Hall exclaimed to the nurse, "Pull, Sally, pull! Put some muscle into it!"

Chapter 9

CHOOSING THE RIGHT OPTION FOR PAIN RELIEF

Choosing the right pain relief option boils down to weighing the benefits of pain relief against the risks of the intervention (Figure 9-1). If pain relief is very important to you, then you will need to compromise on the risks associated with the intervention. If safety is your priority, then you will have to be prepared to tolerate a certain amount of pain. It is a balancing act.

This chapter will walk you through a four-step process to help you make the best decision. You'll need to quietly reflect on your strengths and weaknesses and ascertain which interventions are compatible with your values in life. Your choice must dovetail with your education, upbringing, religion, character, morals, and beliefs. Satisfaction scores from women who have undergone different forms of interventions show that birthing happiness is likely proportional to how consistent the birthing experience was to their expectations. Surprisingly, there is very little correlation between pain relief and satisfaction with the birthing experience; if a woman expects a certain level of pain, then she is likely to not be unsatisfied when it shows up! Ask yourself, is a particular medical intervention congruent with your values? If so, how much is an acceptable intervention? There are no right or wrong answers.

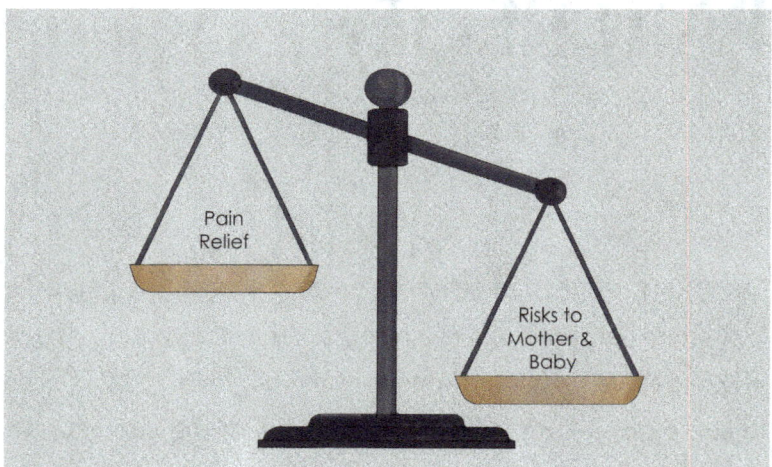

Figure 9-1. The benefits of pain relief must be weighed against the risks of intervention.

Generally speaking, there are two diverse views among women. Some women believe birthing is a natural process and designed perfectly by their Creator, and no human refinement on the process is necessary. They allude to intangible harm that can be caused by meddling with the natural order of things. They argue that what appears to be a quick and easy fix now may be harmful in the long run. Much like hormone replacement therapy was once touted as the fountain of youth in postmenopausal women—only for researchers to discover decades later that it increased the incidence of many forms of cancer—similarly, as we discussed, some studies are pointing to a correlation between autism in children and epidural analgesia. Some studies note lessened psychological bonding between the child and the mother from excessive use of analgesics during labor. Essentially, women with this viewpoint prefer not to intervene with the natural birthing process.

In contrast, many well-informed women want the benefits of current scientific advancements. They're not interested in waiting for future studies to confirm or contradict the current knowledge base. They're ready to make decisions based on what's known now and tacitly consent to address future issues, if any, when they present themselves.

Both views have merits and flaws. What's important is to reflect on your own values and actively participate in your healthcare.

Choosing the right option for pain relief during labor requires careful consideration of several prenatal factors. It's important not to compromise the safety of the baby or the mother in choosing the most effective pain relief. In consultation with your obstetrician, you must consider the following four elements in the course of choosing your desired mode of analgesia:

1. Have there been any problems during your pregnancy?

2. How many times have you given birth previously?

3. What is your level of pain tolerance?

4. Is your choice consistent with your health status, parity, and pain tolerance?

These are the four questions we will walk through, in step, to help you arrive at a decision.

Consider the variables in each step, be honest with your answers, and choose what you feel is best. Understanding how you arrive at your choice is as important as the choice itself.

Step 1. Have there been any problems during your pregnancy?

Determine whether you've had any problems during your pregnancy. If you have had any pregnancy-related complications, you'll be restricted in your choice of labor analgesia. For most patients with pregnancy-related complications, the mode of delivery will be a C-section, preferably under spinal or epidural anesthesia. Sometimes, if the issue is mild or moderate, your obstetrician might suggest a trial of labor. For this trial, an epidural or a continuous spinal may be an excellent choice.

Problems during pregnancy (Figure 9-2) can be broadly classified as those emanating from the baby (fetal) and those emanating from the mother (maternal).

The most common cause of fetus-related difficult labor is the fetal head being too large to travel through the pelvis, which is often referred to as cephalopelvic disproportion. Diabetes during pregnancy can result in a rather large fetus with a pro-portionately large head. It's also expected that if the father is a large individual, he could pass on his genetic traits, resulting in a larger fetus. Rarely, congenital anomalies of the fetus, such as hydrocephalus or tumors, can cause a disproportionately large head on the fetus.

Complications in Pregnancy

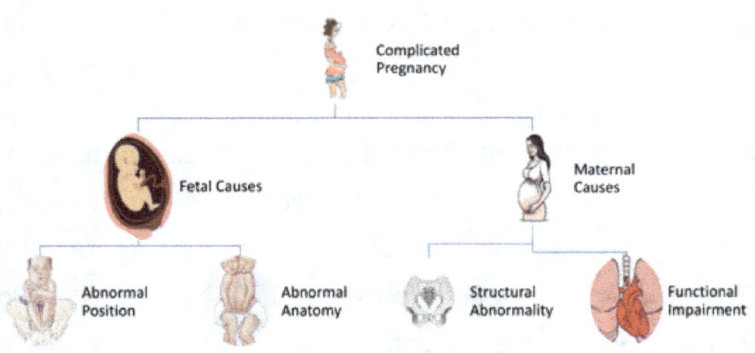

Figure 9-2. Broad classification of complications in pregnancy.

If the cephalopelvic disproportion is minimal, a trial of labor is a possibility to explore. The best pain relief option for this trial of labor is epidural analgesia. During the trial, if the labor pro-gresses well, the baby can be delivered vaginally. Otherwise, the labor either stops or becomes too prolonged. In such situations, the epidural can be deepened or made more of a dense block to permit the obstetrician to perform a cesarean delivery when necessary.

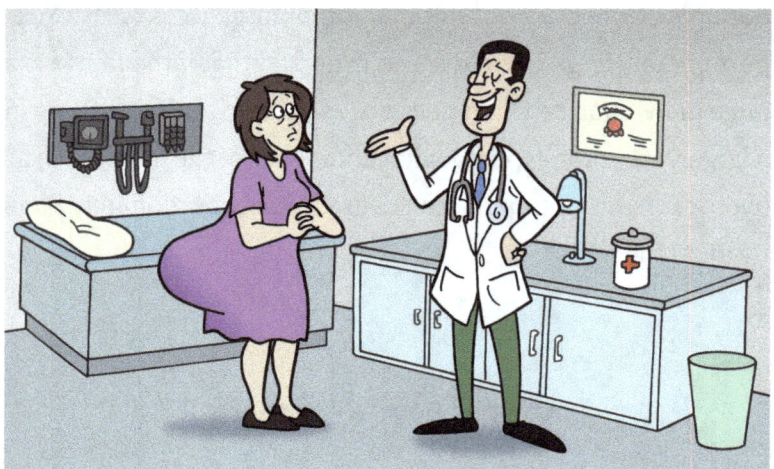

Figure 9-3. "Ms. McKenzie, your son is exploring his habitat; I assure you he will come down by your due date," said Dr. Knowitall.

The second most frequent cause of fetus-related difficult labor is an abnormal presentation of the fetus at the pelvic outlet, meaning the baby is in the wrong position for a smooth birth; this is referred to as fetal malpresentation (Figure 9-3). The two common forms of malpresentation are breech and transverse lie. In breech, the buttocks of the fetus are present at the pelvic outlet instead of the head. In a transverse lie, the fetus is located horizontally to the vertical axis of the uterus, resulting in the back or the side of the fetus presenting at the pelvic outlet.

In nearly half the cases, breech presentation fetuses can be vaginally delivered with no added risk, although some may require cesarean delivery. In contrast, vaginal delivery is rarely possible in a transverse lie fetus. Some obstetricians attempt to convert the fetus to a head-first, or cephalic, presentation by manually pushing the fetus through the patient's abdomen; this is known as the external cephalic version, but it's rarely successful and has the potential to cause significant harm to the fetus. It's often unknown why the fetus has assumed a transverse lie, and applying force risks prematurely dislodging the placenta or compressing the umbilical cord, cutting off oxygen supply to the fetus.

Other rare fetus-related causes for difficult labor include multiple gestations, conjoined fetuses, congenital malformations, hydrocephalus, and tumors of the fetal spine. In most of these circumstances, a planned elective cesarean section under spinal anesthesia is the safest choice for both the mother and the baby.

Maternal causes of complications during pregnancy could include structural abnormalities in the birthing canal or systemic physiological derangements in the mother. Among the structural abnormalities, a small pelvis or deformity of the pelvic ring is often the cause for impeding the passage of the head of the fetus. Sometimes, congenital anomalies of the uterus, cervix, or vagina can prevent the normal passage of the fetus during birth. Existing tumors of the uterus, notably fibroid tumors, can distort the uterine cavity to such an extent that the fetal head would not be able to descend into the birth canal.

Another complication involves the placenta. For unknown reasons, the placenta can attach to the lower segment of the uterus and prevent the fetal head from entering the cervical region, effectively blocking its passage (Figure 9-4).

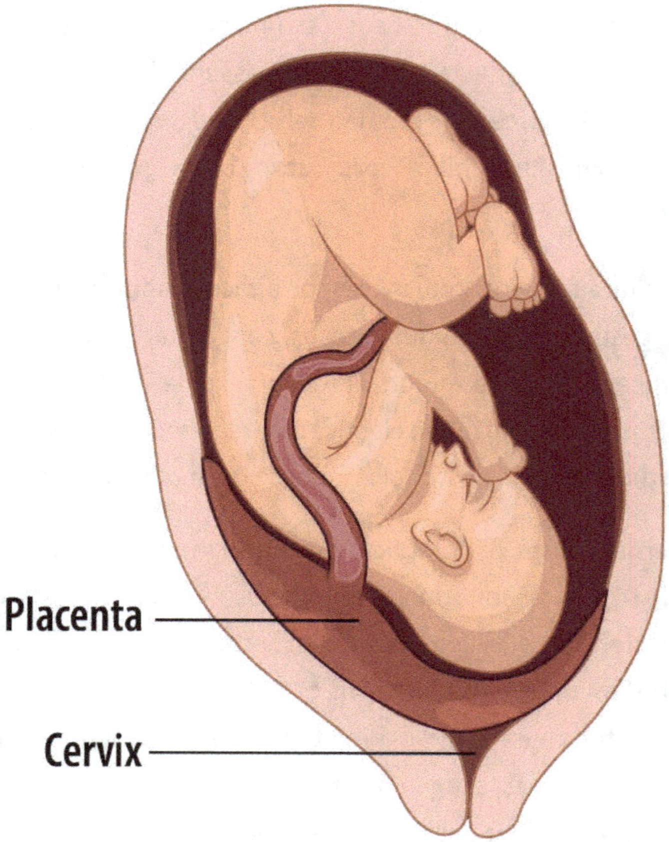

Placenta ——

Cervix ——

Figure 9-4. Abnormal location of the placenta within the uterus (placenta previa).

This condition, known as placenta previa, can lead to cata-strophic bleeding due to premature separation of the placenta from the uterus, which could lead to the death of the fetus, mother, or both. Fortunately, it is relatively easy to identify the location of the placenta on an ultrasound examination, and the best approach in this case is to deliver the baby through a cesarean section.

Functional impairment in the organ systems of the mother is another complication that can have a significant impact on the choice of labor analgesia. Physiological derangements could result from preexisting illnesses such as diabetes, hypertension, and kidney disease, or they could be disorders unique to pregnancy.

Frequently encountered disorders unique to pregnancy include eclampsia, preeclampsia, gestational diabetes, and HELLP syndrome (hemolysis, elevated liver enzymes, and low platelets). In most of these disorders, an uncontrolled rise in blood pressure, along with salt and water retention, could lead to seizures or congestive heart failure. A failing mother's heart could curtail the supply of much-needed nutrients and oxygen to the fetus. Symptoms including hemolysis, elevated liver enzymes, and low platelet count characterize HELLP syndrome. The combination of altered liver function and low platelet counts creates a propensity in the patient to bleed easily and form ineffective blood clots. Bleeding diathesis makes the insertion of an epidural catheter risky. During the insertion of the epidural needle, accidentally puncturing a blood vessel in the spine could lead to an epidural or intrathecal hematoma, which could result in spinal cord or nerve injury with devastating paralysis.

For most patients with systemic disease, a carefully performed epidural is the best choice. If the platelet count is significantly low (under 100,000), as could happen in HELLP syndrome, platelet transfusion should be considered before attempting an epidural. If platelet transfusion is not feasible, a single-shot spinal might be less traumatic, with reduced chances of spinal hematoma formation. Pelvic nerve blocks, in combination with intravenous opioids, can provide reasonable pain relief, particularly in the primigravida.

If a trial of labor has failed, or it is simply too risky to allow the patient to strain for fear of causing heart failure or seizure, an urgent cesarean section should be done to save the fetus and the mother. The vast majority of laboring mothers who fail the trial labor can be safely anesthetized with general anesthesia or spinal anesthesia. General anesthesia takes less time and is often the anesthetic of choice for an emergency cesarean section.

Step 2. How many times have you given birth previously?

The second step is to consider your parity, which is the number of times you've previously given birth. The number of prior births is an important determinant of how painful and protracted your present labor may be.

As shown in Figure 9-5, labor pain becomes less intense in magnitude and duration with subsequent pregnancies. I once met an Iranian mother who was giving birth to her sixth child. She said her pain was less distressing than the cramps she used to experience with her irritable bowel syndrome. She checked into the labor and delivery suite a few minutes past 5:00 p.m. and wanted the baby out before her favorite sitcom began at 7:00

p.m. As she wanted, she pushed with each contraction, and the baby was born in the next 34 minutes! By 7:00 p.m., she was comfortably resting in her hospital bed with her baby on her side, eating supper and watching TV. Her whole labor lasted less than four hours.

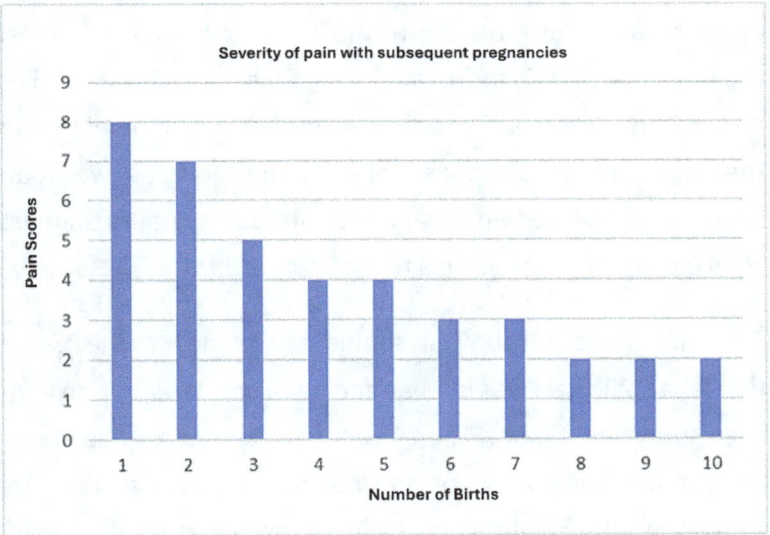

Figure 9-5. Self-reported pain scores of 2,471 Southeast Asian women during subsequent pregnancies.

In contrast, the duration of the first birth in a young mother (under 30 years old) can last from 12 to 24 hours. The historic midwife adage, "She can see one sunrise and one sunset, but never two of either!" is still valid. Unusually long labor, called dystocia, can lead to maternal exhaustion and fetal distress. Failure to progress is one of the most common reasons for C-section in the United States. Dystocia is often the result of unrecognized cephalopelvic disproportion. Prolonged labor may increase the risk of maternal and neonatal infection, fetal distress, neonatal asphyxia, uterine rupture, and postpartum hemorrhage. Instrumented forceps delivery in dystocia may increase the risk of maternal pelvic floor and genital trauma. Such trauma could be the origin for the future development of urinary incontinence and uterine prolapse.

In dystocia, because the uterus must work extra hard to expel the fetus, the pain is more intense and labor is protracted. For this reason, it is essential to receive adequate pain relief during the lengthy and painful phases of stage one and stage two labor. Often, a well-placed epidural or continuous spinal is the best choice for analgesia during a trial of vaginal birth.

From the discussion above, it should now be clear to the reader that labor pain gets less intense and has a shorter duration with each subsequent labor. There are many reasons for this mercy from nature. The primary reason, however, is that the ligaments connecting the pelvic bones become lax and stretched to accommodate the passage of the fetal head.

In addition, the fibromuscular structures, such as the cervix and the vagina, also become farther spread apart and larger in diameter due to stretching and reconfiguration of the elastic connective tissues in them (Figure 9-6). Essentially, the body remembers how it goes the second time around.

Changes in cervical opening

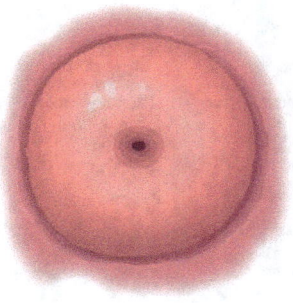

Nulliparous

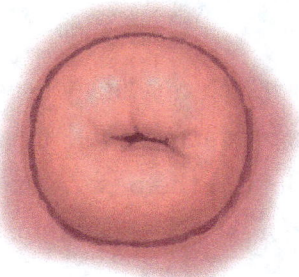

Multiparous

Figure 9-6. Changes in cervical opening with subsequent pregnancies.

Based on the analgesic choice of thousands of women, we can surmise that, for the first pregnancy and labor, an epidural will be the best option (Table 9-1). The pain is often intense, and the labor long. Hence, an effective means of pain relief is necessary. In patients who are obese or have spinal deformities, continuous spinal analgesia is a reasonable alternative to the epidural.

Pregnancy	Gravida 1, 2, 3	Gravida 4, 5	Gravida 6 and Greater
Pain intensity	High	Moderate	Low
Type of analgesia	Epidural Continuous spinal Combined spinal epidural (CSE)	Single shot spinal Paracervical block Pudendal nerve block Nitrous oxide IV opioids	Natural birth Lamaze Water birth Hypnosis Acupuncture Nitrous oxide IV opioids

Table 9-1. Recommended types of analgesia based on gravida.

Gravidas 2 and 3 will also very likely experience significant pain and somewhat protracted labor. Here again, an epidural or a continuous spinal is the best choice. The risk-benefit ratio is still in favor of these interventions.

Gravidas 4 and 5 do not require a continuous pain relief modality such as epidural or continuous spinal analgesia. Inserting a catheter tilts the risk-benefit ratio, not in favor of the epidural or continuous spinal. A single intrathecal injection, often called a single shot spinal, will be more than adequate to cover the later painful parts of stage one and stage two labor. A carefully timed single shot spinal should provide two to three hours of pain relief. If, for some reason, the labor is protracted, the obstetrician should be able to supplement the spinal with a paracervical block or pudendal nerve block to aid the delivery of the baby in stage two. Breathing nitrous oxide or intravenous Demerol, morphine, or fentanyl would also greatly supplement the pain relief from the spinal.

Gravidas 6 and greater often do not require any form of spinal interventions or pelvic blocks. The pain intensity is significantly diminished, and the labor is often quick and precipitous. If necessary, intravenous opioids, such as nalbuphine or butorphanol, can be used to provide pain relief and sedation. Here, you could also try nonpharmacological pain relief and coping measures such as Lamaze, water birth, acupuncture, hypnosis, and other natural birth measures discussed in Chapter 8. All drugs, whether they're local anesthetics, intravenous opioids, or nitrous oxide, pose a measurable risk of danger to the mother and child, allowing for many tangible benefits to a "drug-free" birthing. The risk-benefit ratio strongly favors fewer pharmaceutical interventions in women giving birth to their sixth or later child.

Step 3. What is your level of pain tolerance?

Step 3 involves understanding your level of pain tolerance. You must candidly ask yourself, "How much pain can I tolerate for six or seven hours?" For comparison, in your first pregnancy, the labor will likely be protracted 10 to 12 hours. Use the illustration in Figure 9-7 to help you determine how intense your pain is likely to be and whether you have the mental fortitude to go through several hours of this magnitude of pain if you are contemplating a natural birth.

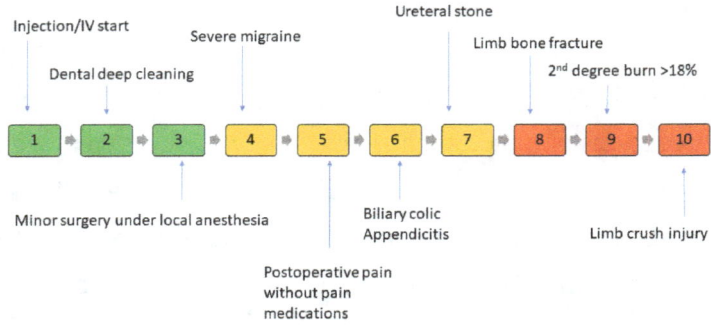

Figure 9-7. Different types of pain generators and their pain severity scores.

Most mothers going through their first labor report the peak intensity of labor pain to be between seven and eight on a zero to 10 pain scale. If there's any degree of cephalopelvic disproportion, the pain increases to an eight or nine. If the baby is small or the mother's pelvis is roomy, the pain often decreases to a six or seven. Most multiparous women who have had three or more prior births report pain in the range of four to seven.

It's not uncommon for first-time mothers to give natural birth a trial run for several hours before asking for an epidural. There's nothing wrong with this strategy but be mindful that complications from the epidural itself increase if it's attempted in later phases of the first stage of labor. When the cervix is 8 to 10 centimeters dilated, the contractions are often intense and repeated every one to two minutes. In this situation, you will not be able to sit or lie still for the anesthesiologist to place the epidural safely. It will be the difference between shooting a running deer and one standing still. You'll be subjecting yourself to all the risks of an epidural for only a few hours of benefit. Thus, if you're obese, suffer from edema due to toxemia of pregnancy or spinal deformities such as scoliosis, or you've had prior spine surgery, you should opt to request an epidural earlier rather than later. This will give the anesthesiologist sufficient unhurried time to place the epidural.

There's a spectrum of pain relief options to consider based on your level of pain tolerance, whether this is your first birth or not (Figure 9-8).

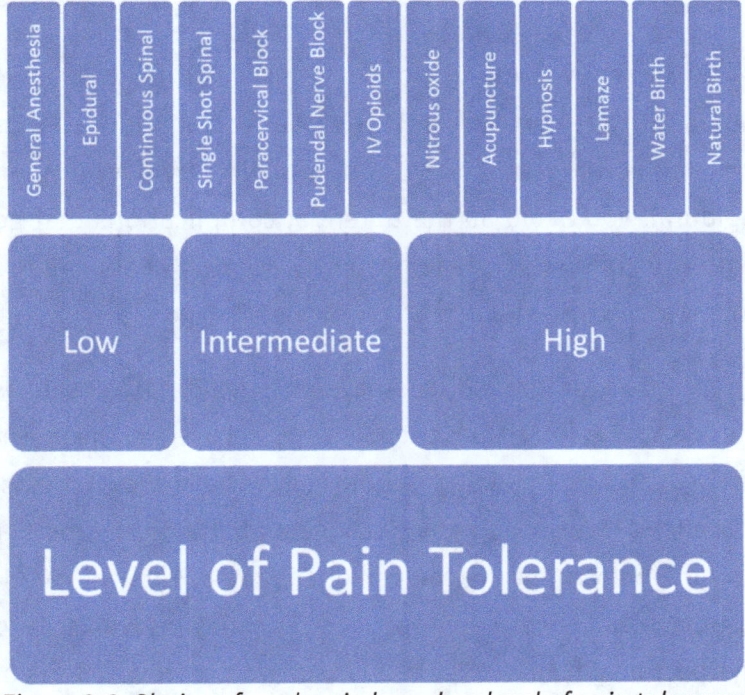

Figure 9-8. Choice of analgesia based on level of pain tolerance.

If your pain tolerance is low, you're better off with an epidural or continuous spinal analgesia. If you would describe yourself as having intermediate pain tolerance, located somewhere between low pain tolerance and high pain tolerance, your best choice is to try a single shot spinal. This might be combined with paracervical or pudendal nerve blocks to increase the quality and duration of analgesia.

If you feel your pain tolerance is high, then you might opt for intravenous pain medications or inhalation of nitrous oxide gas. Nonpharmaceutical options such as hypnosis, acupuncture, water birth, and Lamaze might also be appropriate for you.

At this stage, you might wonder if it's worth foregoing the epidural. The short answer is yes. The long answer depends on what's important to you in your life. By avoiding an epidural, you avoid all the potential complications that go with the epidural. More importantly, we don't know all the long-term adverse effects of epidurals.

For example, as we've discussed, some well-designed studies show a strong correlation between epidural use and the prevalence of autism. In addition, some studies have shown the occurrence of weak or dysthymic bonding between the mother and the baby following the use of epidurals. The lack of adequate bonding may, in later years, manifest as broken and dysfunctional families. These two important adverse effects of epidurals are often downplayed or discredited by the medical-pharmaceutical industrial complex. There is an enormous financial benefit to the medical system in offering epidurals to all laboring mothers.

In contrast, there is minimal incentive to favor natural birth. The epidural makes the patient happy, it reduces the demand on the obstetrician, rewards the anesthesiologist, and pharmaceutical companies get to sell more drugs. There's no money in withholding an epidural.

On the other hand, by avoiding an epidural, you will have to determine whether any other pain relief option is a good fit for you during childbirth. Avoiding all labor pain relief options is not always in the best interest of the laboring mother. Assessing your pain tolerance is an excellent step toward understanding how best to support yourself through childbirth.

Step 4. Is your choice consistent with health status, parity, and pain tolerance?

Let us put all the preceding information together and create a pain management plan. The flow chart in Figure 9-9 can help you walk through each element to consider when determining which choice is best for you.

In deciding your choice of labor pain relief, the first question to ask is whether the pregnancy is normal. Problems with the pregnancy may arise from the fetus or the mother. Some of these abnormalities might be minimal, and vaginal birth may still be an option. Hence, a follow-up question should be asked: is your obstetrician planning on a trial of labor? If a trial of labor is planned, then an epidural, continuous spinal, or combined spinal-epidural is your best option. Should the trial of labor fail, as evidenced by prolonged labor and fetal or maternal distress, the existing epidural catheter can be used to quickly deepen the block and convert the epidural analgesia into epidural anesthesia. This is usually accomplished by injecting a higher concentration of local anesthetic (Table 9-2). If time is of the essence, then rapidly acting local anesthetics must be chosen [49].

LOCAL ANESTHETIC	DOSE	ONSET OF ANESTHESIA
2-Chloroprocaine 3%	20 ml	14 minutes
Lidocaine 2% with 1:200,000 epinephrine	20 ml	16 minutes
Ropivacaine 0.75%	20 ml	18 minutes
Bupivacaine 0.5%	20 ml	20 minutes

Table 9-2. Commonly used local anesthetics to convert epidural analgesia into anesthesia.

If the abnormalities are severe and a trial of labor and vaginal birth could be dangerous, then your obstetrician will likely plan on an elective cesarean section. The surgery is usually scheduled close to the expected date of delivery. A spinal anesthesia is the best option for an elective cesarean section. A spinal anesthesia requires only a very small amount of local anesthetic to be injected into the spine, and the mother remains awake. There is little transfer of medications through the placenta to the fetus, and the baby is born awake and alert. The mother can participate in the birthing process, provide immediate skin-to-skin contact with the baby, and vocalize emotions, strengthening the bond between the mother and the baby.

If there are fetal or maternal abnormalities and you're in active labor, or there is fetal or maternal distress because of the abnormalities, then an emergency cesarean may be indicated. Because time is of the essence to prevent harm to the mother or the baby, general anesthesia is usually preferred. It takes far less time to render the patient unconscious than an epidural or spinal. Often, the baby can be delivered in a matter of minutes. The fastest cesarean section I have witnessed was seven minutes, including the time it took to anesthetize the patient and perform the surgery to deliver the baby. The downside to general anesthesia is that the baby is often born depressed and anesthetized by the general anesthetics traversing the placenta and reaching the baby in the minutes before delivery.

If, on the other hand, your pregnancy has been normal, with no fetal or maternal abnormalities, then you must ask yourself, "What's my level of pain tolerance?"

Irrespective of the number of prior labors, if your pain tolerance is low, then you'll be better served with an epidural, continuous spinal, or combined spinal epidural (CSE). One way to objectively assess your pain tolerance is to reach back into your past experience and recall how distressing certain medical procedures were. For example, if placing an intravenous catheter, or dental cleaning, or minor skin procedures under local anesthesia were painful and distressing to you, then you probably have low pain tolerance.

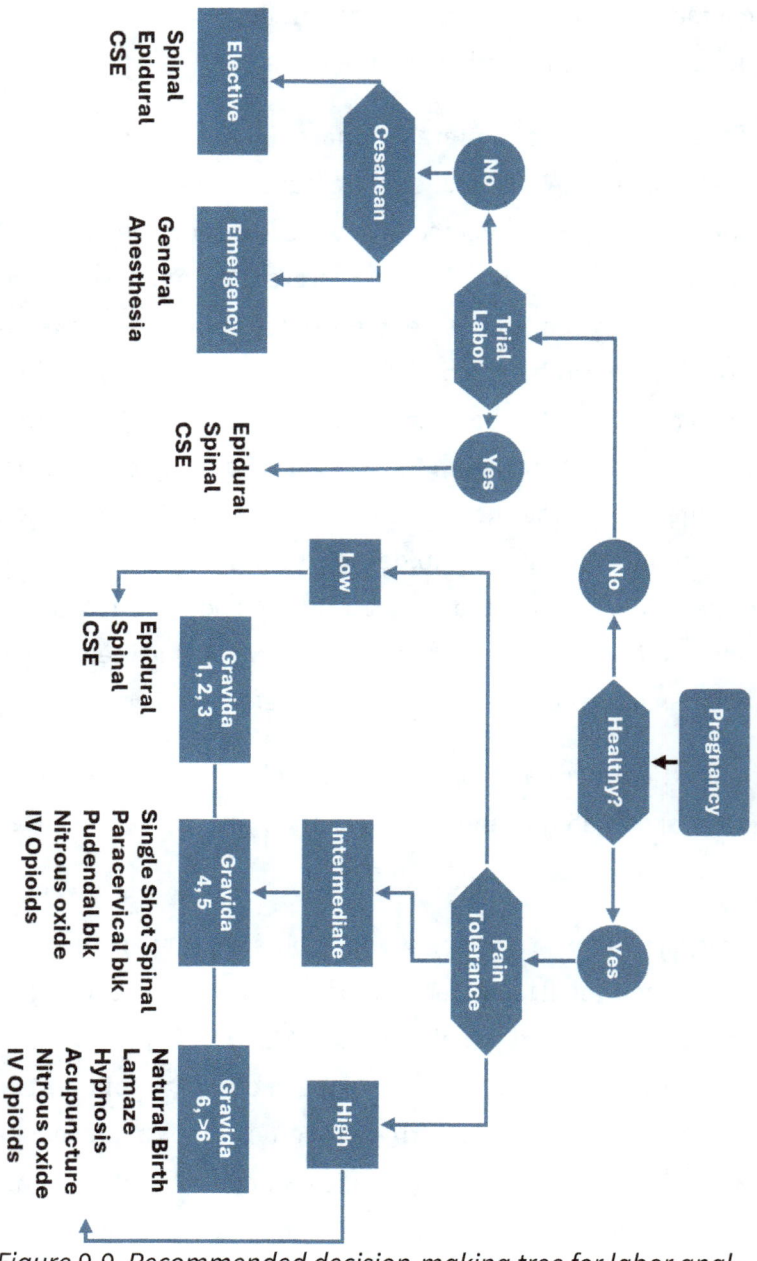

Figure 9-9. Recommended decision-making tree for labor analgesia.

Even though labor gets less painful with each subsequent birth, you're better off with the predictable pain relief provided by an epidural, continuous spinal, or CSE.

However, if your pain tolerance is high, you should consider opting to minimize medical intervention and go with a more natural childbirth.

As discussed previously, minimal interventions include no medications, Lamaze, hypnosis, acupuncture, water birth, IV opioids, and nitrous oxide. Again, to determine if you have high pain tolerance, consider how you felt following a previous painful incident such as a major surgery, a long bone fracture, a second-degree burn to greater than 18 percent of your body, or a crush injury to your limbs. Even though these injuries are excruciating, if you were able to tolerate them, it's likely you have a high pain tolerance and will do just fine with minimal medical intervention to mitigate your labor pain.

If you aren't sure of your pain tolerance, it's best to align with the average. Most women have an intermediate level of pain tolerance. Even though it's painful, they can tolerate severe migraines, postoperative pain, appendicitis, biliary colic, ureteral colic, or large deep lacerations without pain medications. For these women, an epidural is often not necessary, and in this situation, the number of prior labors is helpful in deciding the best pain relief options for women with intermediate levels of pain tolerance.

- Gravidas 1, 2, and 3 ⇒ epidural, continuous spinal, or CSE

- Gravidas 4 and 5 ⇒ single shot spinal, paracervical block, pudendal block, IV opioids, nitrous oxide

- Gravidas 6 or more ⇒ natural birth, Lamaze, hypnosis, acupuncture, water birth, IV opioids, nitrous oxide

The recommendations above show that the first three labors are generally the most painful experiences. However, the pain improves with subsequent labor; hence, less intervention is necessary.

In summary, if your pregnancy has been healthy with no fetal abnormalities or maternal abnormalities, and you have a low pain tolerance, your choice should be an epidural or continuous spinal or CSE. On the contrary, if you have a high pain tolerance, you should minimize spinal interventions and opt for a more natural childbirth. It is still reasonable to supplement your natural birth with intravenous pain medications or breathing nitrous oxide. If your pain tolerance is intermediate, then for the first three pregnancies, you will be better advised to opt for an epidural or continuous spinal or CSE. If it is your fourth or fifth pregnancy, you may opt for a single-shot spinal, paracervical block, or pudendal nerve block. Finally, if it is your sixth or later pregnancy, you are better off foregoing any form of spinal intervention and opting for more natural childbirth. Natural childbirth options can be supplemented with intravenous pain medications or nitrous oxide as necessary during the course of labor.

If your pregnancy has been complicated by maternal or fetal abnormalities, then your obstetrician may advise an elective cesarean section. This is best achieved under spinal anesthesia.

If your obstetrician suggests a trial of labor, then an epidural or continuous spinal, or CSE are your best options.

Study the decision-making tree shown in Figure 9-9 carefully and discuss it with all concerned parties—your obstetrician, partner, friends, and family. Everyone is slightly different in their physical constitution and mental and emotional makeup. Hence, the structure of the decision tree will need to be modified to accommodate for individual variations and feedback that you receive from others.

In Appendix II, I have included a template for creating a birth plan. Once you've decided on the best pain relief method, this is a good place to document your preferences for labor and delivery and tactfully convey that information to your obstetrician and other hospital providers. Feel free to copy or remove those pages to create your plan.

Chapter 10

FREQUENTLY ASKED QUESTIONS

This chapter serves as a quick reference for frequently asked questions about labor analgesia. While much of this information is covered in greater detail in other chapters, you can consult those sections for more in-depth explanations of specific techniques or to locate relevant medical literature on a topic. The answers provided here are intended to be concise and will guide you toward more comprehensive discussions on the subject.

What will labor be like without pain medications or epidurals?

Most women describe labor as one of the most painful experiences of their lives. However, the intensity of labor pain tends to decrease with each subsequent birth. One mother who had her first baby without any pain medications or an epidural compared the pain to that of a broken ankle she suffered while hiking and had to walk back a few miles to seek help. Another mother likened it to the pain of a kidney stone. In contrast, a mother who had her fifth child described the experience as merely uncomfortable, similar to colic. It's important to remember that humanity has existed for millions of years without the aid of epidurals and has managed well. Even today, 70 percent of the world's population does not have access to labor analgesia and experiences labor without significant adverse outcomes.

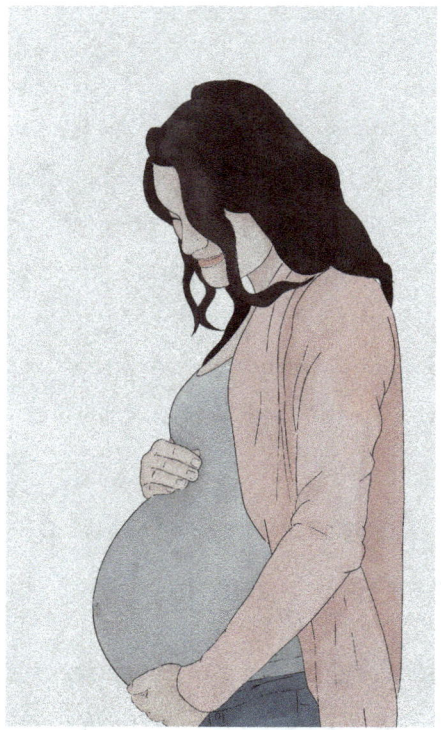

Figure 10-1. Knowing what to expect during pregnancy and labor will help alleviate stress and improve outcomes.

What pain-relief options are available to control labor pain?

Epidural analgesia is the most frequently utilized pain relief method for women in Western countries. It's highly effective and predictable in relieving pain. This might be an excellent choice for many women, particularly if they're having their first or second babies. However, it comes with numerous potential short- and long-term complications. The risk of these complications must be weighed against the temporary relief of pain and your priorities in life.

Spinal analgesia (intrathecal injection) is another excellent option for women in the later stages of labor. Spinal analgesia also carries a similar complication profile to epidural and should be opted for after careful deliberation of its complications.

Nerve blocks, such as pudendal or paracervical blocks, can be quickly performed by your obstetrician. They provide a somewhat lesser quality of pain relief and are often unpredictable in their outcomes. The pudendal block will anesthetize the perineum but provide a lesser degree of relief from uterine contractions.

Intravenous opioid pain medications are a good option for women who do not want epidurals, spinals, or nerve blocks. Although qualitatively less effective in controlling labor pain, they do offer moderate pain relief and blunt the intensity of strong uterine contraction pain. The downside to any intravenous pain medication is that the medication will travel through the bloodstream and reach the child within the uterus. Often, the child will be born sedated and have difficulty breathing, or have a slow heart rate and low blood pressure.

Inhaling nitrous oxide is another excellent pain relief option for some women. Breathing nitrous oxide blunts the intensity of uterine contraction pain. It can be used intermittently as needed, thus minimizing hypoxia in the fetus. However, the pain relief is often inadequate and unpredictable.

General anesthesia is often the last resort to terminate acute, unabated pain, particularly if the fetus is stuck at the outlet and cannot be delivered without the assistance of forceps or a vacuum extractor.

Nonpharmacological pain relief methods—yoga, hypnosis, acupuncture, water birth, massage, doula-provided continuous support, Lamaze, and so on—are often less effective in controlling pain but have no significant complications or side effects on the mother or the child. These methods are best utilized by well-motivated and strong-willed mothers who practice them before the actual day of labor.

How is an epidural or spinal performed?

An epidural or spinal anesthesia is typically performed while you are either sitting up or lying on your side. It can be helpful to position yourself by tucking your chin to your chest, relaxing your shoulders, and curling up by bringing your knees toward your abdomen. This position, known as the "fetal position," resembles how a fetus is curled inside the uterus. It creates more space between your vertebrae, making it easier for your anesthesiologist to access the epidural or intrathecal space in your lower back.

The procedure begins with the anesthesiologist injecting a local anesthetic into the skin of your lower back to numb a small area. They will then use a special needle to gently advance into the epidural or intrathecal space in your spine. Following this, a tiny plastic catheter is inserted through the needle and into the spine before the needle is removed. Once the anesthesiologist confirms that the catheter is in the correct position, they will inject pain medication through it. The spinal catheter is often secured to your back with tape, and a continuous infusion of pain medication will be administered throughout your labor until the delivery of your baby.

When is an epidural or spinal performed?

The epidural is often performed in stage one of labor when the cervix is three to four centimeters dilated and the uterine contractions are strong and regular. A single shot spinal can be performed much later in the labor when the cervix is eight to nine centimeters dilated. However, the longer one waits, the more difficult it becomes to sit still or lie down comfortably without moving during the procedure. Excessive movements make it difficult for the anesthesiologist to properly access the epidural or spinal space, which is akin to shooting a moving target. If you cannot sit or lie still for the procedure, your complications may increase.

How long does it take to perform an epidural or spinal?

The epidural generally takes about 30 minutes to perform. If your spine is deformed or if you're obese, then the procedure could take up to an hour to achieve the desired result. There are circumstances, such as morbid obesity, edema, spinal deformities (e.g., scoliosis or kyphosis), or prior spine surgery, when it's nearly impossible to achieve a satisfactory epidural or spinal analgesia. Persistent attempts under these conditions could lead to more complications and catastrophic adverse events. If you have any of these conditions, you and your obstetrician must discuss all analgesic options with your anesthesiologist before your due date.

How will the epidural or spinal make me feel?

You will feel numb below the level of your ribcage. Your lower limbs—feet, legs, and thighs—will feel weak. You might not be able to control them. You will still feel the dull pressure of the fetal head. Often, blood pressure drops initially due to profound vasodilation and blood pooling in the lower limbs and pelvis. This is easily corrected with an IV fluid bolus and pressure medications. When the pressure drops, mothers complain of light-headedness and nausea. These symptoms abate once the blood pressure returns to normal.

Do I have to stay in bed after an epidural or spinal?

Yes, it would be best if you stayed in bed after an epidural or spinal. Your leg muscles will be weak, and there's a real chance of falling and hurting yourself and the baby. This is why we often recommend that mothers use the bathroom to empty their bladder and bowels before starting an epidural or spinal.

Can I have a "walking epidural"?

Yes, you can, but I wouldn't recommend it. The "walking epidural" is a technique where a very dilute solution of local anesthetic mixed with an opioid is infused into the epidural space to preferentially block the pain sensation without affecting the motor and other sensory nerves.

In theory, the "walking epidural" sounds great; you can walk and receive pain relief at the same time. In reality, you get neither pain relief nor guaranteed safety while walking. In my 40-plus years of experience, I have rarely seen this technique provide adequate pain relief to mothers. It's somewhat of an aspirational hype, yet it has found a niche in the pantheons of medical literature and continues to live in medical journals and textbooks.

If you need to walk a short distance after the epidural, always ask for two-person assistance. One person on each side should be holding you. First, dangle your legs on the side of the bed to make sure you can move them and control them, then stand by the bedside and see if your legs are strong enough to hold your weight. If you don't feel lightheaded and your legs are strong enough to hold your weight, with two-person assistance, you may walk short distances. The nurse should make sure you're not going to pull out your epidural or the IV line.

Can I eat after an epidural or spinal?

It's generally advisable not to eat solid food after an epidural or spinal. You should drink clear liquids like water, soda, non-pulp fruit juice, black coffee, tea, or clear broth.

If your labor is not progressing well and your obstetrician is considering a cesarean section, or you're obese, diabetic, or suffer from obstructive sleep apnea, then you should consider stopping all oral intake at least two hours before the anticipated cesarean or vaginal delivery.

Historically, measures to prevent aspiration of stomach contents into the lungs have been the single most important advancements in reducing maternal death around labor and delivery.

Are there any adverse effects to epidural or spinal analgesia?

Yes, there are several potential adverse effects related to epidural or spinal analgesia. Here are some of the more common ones.

There's a decrease in blood pressure. This occurs due to the profound vasodilation in your lower limbs and pelvis secondary to the blockade of the sympathetic nervous system. Fluid bolus or vasopressor medications, such as ephedrine or phenylephrine, can reverse this.

Decreases in heart rate are primarily due to the paralysis of the sympathetic nerves that supply your heart. If left uncorrected, they could lead to low blood pressure or cardiac arrest. Fortunately, this is easily correctable with medications such as atropine or epinephrine.

You may experience shortness of breath. This is due to the weakness of the abdominal and lower intercostal muscles necessary for breathing. In most patients, this can be corrected by simply elevating the head of the bed and providing supplemental oxygen to the mother. Rarely, the epidural infusion may have to be stopped or decreased to lower the level of the spinal anesthesia.

Another serious complication is total paralysis, also called a "total spinal," which occurs when a local anesthetic bolus is accidentally injected into the intrathecal space instead of the spine's epidural space. Although rare in the hands of experienced anesthesiologists, this complication does occur with some regularity in teaching hospitals. All four limbs, as well as the abdominal and chest muscles, are paralyzed by the local anesthetic, which is now mixed with the cerebrospinal fluid. You will feel numb below the level of your neck. You cannot move your limbs, breathe, or speak when this happens. A profound decrease in blood pressure and heart rate often accompanies this. This is a medical emergency and should be recognized promptly and treated immediately. Survival will depend on prompt intubation of your trachea and initiation of mechanical ventilation. In addition, fluids, vasopressors, and inotropic agents might be needed to resuscitate the heart and blood pressure. The paralysis will resolve once the effects of the local anesthetic wear off.

Spinal headaches can occur in one to six percent of patients who undergo spinal or epidural anesthesia. However, if the outer layer of the membranes covering the spinal cord, known as the dura mater, is accidentally punctured during the placement of an epidural with an 18G or 17G needle, the chances of developing a spinal headache increase to nearly 50 percent. These headaches can start immediately or may be delayed for a few days before they appear. They typically present as a throbbing or aching pain felt in the forehead, sides, and back of the head. Symptoms worsen when the patient stands up, sits up, sneezes, or coughs. Accompanying symptoms may include nausea and vomiting. Although rare, some patients may experience involvement of the cranial nerves, leading to double vision or ringing in the ears. Fortunately, spinal headaches are usually self-limiting and tend to resolve after a few days with symptomatic treatment. Most patients find relief through rest, hydration, and the use of non-steroidal anti-inflammatory drugs (NSAIDs). In severe cases, an epidural blood patch may be required to alleviate the symptoms.

Some women experience persistent lower back pain following an epidural or spinal. However, it's tough to differentiate whether the pain was caused by the mechanical forces of labor acting on a lax spine and pelvic girdle or injury to ligaments, membranes, and nerves caused by the epidural or spinal needle. Fortunately, the back pain resolves over time as the pregnancy hormones recede and normal hormonal levels are established over several weeks to months.

In a few patients in one or both lower limbs, a sensation of numbness, tingling, or sharp pain may be experienced for several months or permanently following an epidural or spinal. This pain is thought to result from the needle lacerating a nerve or the catheter causing nerve contusion. In rare cases, the damage could be permanent if the local anesthetic is injected into a nerve (intraneural injection).

The epidural needle or the catheter can accidentally puncture or lacerate an artery or vein in the spine and cause bleeding. The bleeding can be outside the spinal dura (epidural) or within the dura (sub-dural). When this happens, the collecting blood or hematoma can compress the spinal nerves or the spinal cord, resulting in paralysis. The most dangerous version of compression is cauda equina syndrome in which the nerve roots in the lower part of the spinal cord are compressed by an expanding hematoma, resulting in numbness in the perineum, weakness in lower limbs, and loss of bladder and bowel control. This is a surgical emergency and will require immediate spinal decompression and control of the bleeding. Spinal bleeding is more likely to occur in women with excessive bleeding tendencies.

Bacteria from the skin surface or contaminated needle or catheter can be driven into the deeper tissues of the spine.

Spreading infection can cause skin infection, meningitis, or myelitis.

Brown-Sequard syndrome is a rare condition that occurs from repeated and traumatic attempts at placement of an epidural or spinal at the upper lumbar or lower thoracic region of the spine. It's a partial injury to one side of the spinal cord, resulting in weakness in one lower limb and loss of pain and temperature sensations in the other limb. If the injury resulted from a contusion from the needle or catheter, symptoms often resolve in a few days. However, if the segmental arteries that supply the spinal cord (artery of Adamkiewicz) are severed, then full recovery might not be possible.

Will the epidural have any adverse effects on my labor?

Even though most obstetricians and anesthesiologists minimize or downplay the adverse effects of epidurals on labor, there are some critical adverse consequences to epidurals to consider.

First, prolongation of labor can occur. Nearly all the studies that have looked into the duration of labor have uniformly concluded stage one of labor is prolonged by epidurals. In my experience, an epidural can prolong the total duration you will be in labor, including stages two and three. And while it's no picnic to have your labor experience prolonged, additional complications can occur with longer labor. Generally speaking, the longer the labor lasts, the greater the chances of uterine infection, fever, exhaustion, and other adverse effects on the mother.

With an epidural, there can be an increased need for oxytocin infusion. Because the progression of labor slows down with epidurals, most obstetricians will start an infusion of oxytocin to stimulate the uterus. Oxytocin can cause nausea, vomiting, fluid retention, and excessive stimulation of the uterus. In patients with uterine scars, such as from previous cesarean sections or fibroid surgery, this can lead to uterine rupture and the death of the baby.

An epidural can result in increased use of forceps. The epidural temporarily weakens the lower abdominal and pelvic muscles, making it difficult for laboring mothers to strain and push the baby out. Often the head remains stuck at the vaginal outlet without much movement. This is when most obstetricians apply the outlet forceps to deliver the baby. It is also a customary practice for nurses to push on the patient's lower abdomen to assist in the expulsion of the baby. The forceps can cause significant trauma to the baby's skull, brain, ears, nose, eyes, and facial bones. They also increase the chances of perineal tears and the use of episiotomies.

The epidural slows the descent of the fetal head and opening of the uterine cervix and thus can result in a prolonged stage one labor, leading to an increased need for unplanned cesarean sections. Prolonged labor, also termed "failure to progress," is often cited as the reason for performing cesarean sections. Cesarean sections come with all the risks and complications of anesthesia and surgery.

Will the epidural affect my baby?

Even though the risk is small, an epidural can negatively affect your baby. The risks can be immediate or delayed. For example, fetal distress is often an immediate adverse event in the baby. It is characterized by the slowing of the fetal heart rate and the onset of acidosis in the baby. This is due to a lack of sufficient oxygen in the fetal circulation, which stems from a decreased amount of oxygen reaching the placenta due to maternal low blood pressure and heart rate as a result of the epidural. This is called hypoxemia, which can be further worsened by poor ventilation of the mother due to the weakening of the abdominal and lower intercostal muscles.

If the oxygen deprivation to the fetus is not corrected promptly, certain parts of the brain will suffer cell death, also called apoptosis (e.g., periventricular leukomalacia). This will manifest as cerebral palsy a few days to a few months or even years after birth. This could affect the child's body movements and walking control or lead to cognitive impairment, epilepsy, defective vision, and hearing. Astonishingly, most medical textbooks do not mention epidurals as a potential causative factor in the development of cerebral palsy.

Additionally, several population-based studies show a strong correlation between autism and the use of epidurals. The specific mechanisms of injury are unclear at this time; however, it is likely related to deprivation of oxygen to the fetal brain. It could also be related to the toxicity of drugs used in the epidural. The diagnosis may not be evident immediately after birth, and the symptoms could take a few years to manifest. Difficulty with social interactions, repetitive behaviors, attention deficits, hyperactivity, impaired learning, and anxiety are often the early symptoms.

What is the best alternative to an epidural or spinal?

All pain relief options come with certain risks. In my opinion, the second-best choice after an epidural or spinal anesthesia is intravenous opioid medications. An example of this is remifentanil, which can be administered as patient-controlled analgesia (PCA). This could be complemented by a paracervical block provided by your obstetrician. It's important to remember that natural childbirth should always remain an option.

Is natural childbirth safe?

Natural childbirth is generally considered safe, with very few fetal or maternal conditions that would prevent it. Your obstetrician can identify any potential issues during prenatal care and advise you on your options. In many medical situations, allowing the natural physiological process to proceed with minimal intervention often results in better outcomes. Monitoring the mother's vital signs and the baby's heart rate adds an important layer of safety. The obstetrician must remain vigilant and be ready to intervene if there are any signs of distress for either the mother or the baby. One of the challenges of natural childbirth is the significant pain that can accompany it. Approximately 60 percent of women who initially plan for a natural birth eventually request some form of pain relief during labor. Success in achieving a natural birth can depend on several factors, including pain tolerance, the number of previous births, any existing medical conditions, motivation, physical stamina, social support, and the medical staff's attitude toward natural childbirth.

Chapter 11

THE 10 KEYS TO A GREAT BIRTHING EXPERIENCE

In my practice as an anesthesiologist, I've had the privilege of caring for a diverse array of patients during pregnancy and childbirth. The women who had peaceful pregnancies and joyous births often had a clear understanding of certain foundational principles. They spoke up for themselves and asserted their choices.

I've distilled here the key elements that make the difference between a great birthing experience and a disastrous chain of uncontrolled events leading to the birth of your child. I refer to these core elements as the "keys to a great birthing experience." This holistic framework will equip you with the knowledge, confidence, and support systems needed to navigate this incredible rite of passage with grace, positivity, and a profound sense of personal power. As such, this is an excellent framework to help you make the best choices for your childbirth experience.

1. Childbirth is natural.

The female body is designed such that childbirth can occur vaginally without any medical intervention. The fact that humanity has existed for millions of years and increased in population is a testament to the strength and efficiency of this design. No one *needs* an epidural. No harm will occur because of the lack of labor analgesia. In my medical practice of over 40 years, I have never seen a single case of complications due to a *lack* of pain medication. Of the approximately 140 million deliveries worldwide yearly, no more than 10 percent get any form of labor analgesia. If you were born before 1990, there is a very good chance your mother did not have an epidural; she survived, and you turned out okay. The rates for analgesic intervention are far higher in the United States and Europe, reaching 60 to 80 percent, depending upon the race of the parturient. But this does not mean a painless birth is better than a natural birth. Because childbirth is such a natural process, and because the female body is designed to manage through it without pain control, it is vitally important to avoid over-treatment. More medical care is not necessarily better in this case.

2. Be prepared for the day of birthing.

You have nearly nine months to plan for this day. Think through all the activities that need to be well-synchronized for you to transition from home to the hospital and back with the baby. When the contractions start, who will drive you to the hospital? What about if you need to go in at 2 a.m.? What items will you take with you to the hospital? Do you have clothing for the baby? Do you have a car seat to bring the baby home safely? Who will stay with you at the hospital? Who will watch your home when you're gone? Do you have other children who need caretaking while you're in the hospital? It's fun to read in the news how the taxi driver or the police officer delivered a baby in the backseat of a car, but you don't want to be that person if you can help it. It's too risky.

3. Get fit before birthing.

Labor is a physically and emotionally challenging process. It would be best if you were physically, emotionally, and spiritually prepared for it. Give up harmful substances like alcohol, smoking, and recreational drugs. During pregnancy, just as in a well-lived life, good nutrition, adequate exercise, and plenty of rest are essential for your physical well-being. If you suffer from preeclampsia, diabetes, or high blood pressure, make sure to take your prescribed medications to keep your physiology close to normal. For emotional health, avoid negative individuals. Stay away from activities that provoke anxiety or depression. If you practice a religion, seek out guidance and blessings for you and the baby through your faith. Women who are physically and emotionally fit go through labor with minimal adverse events and report positive, enriching, and affirmative experiences.

4. Doulas make a positive difference in your birthing experience.

While it's nice to have a partner or other close person with you during the labor and birth of your baby, having an experienced professional there can bring an additional level of comfort and confidence to the process. However, be mindful that most hospital staff will not be able to fill that role adequately. Your nurse, for instance, will be too busy changing your IV, putting on the monitors, and typing notes on the computer. Rarely will they stay with you during your contractions; the good ones might, but most will not be able to. Your obstetrician will visit periodically to monitor your progress, but will not participate in getting you through the painful contractions.

In contrast, a good doula will stay with you for the entire duration of the labor and offer continuous emotional and physical support. They will talk to you, hold your hand, massage your belly, assist you with breathing, and get you through the most demanding and painful parts of your labor. If you're financially able or if your insurance will cover the costs, engage the services of a good doula early in your pregnancy. Studies show that a doula's presence decreases labor length, significantly decreases the need for cesarean sections, and results in less use of pain medications and higher rates of breastfeeding. In many Asian and African cultures, doulas have been an integral part of birthing for centuries (Figure 11-1). They're worth their weight in gold.

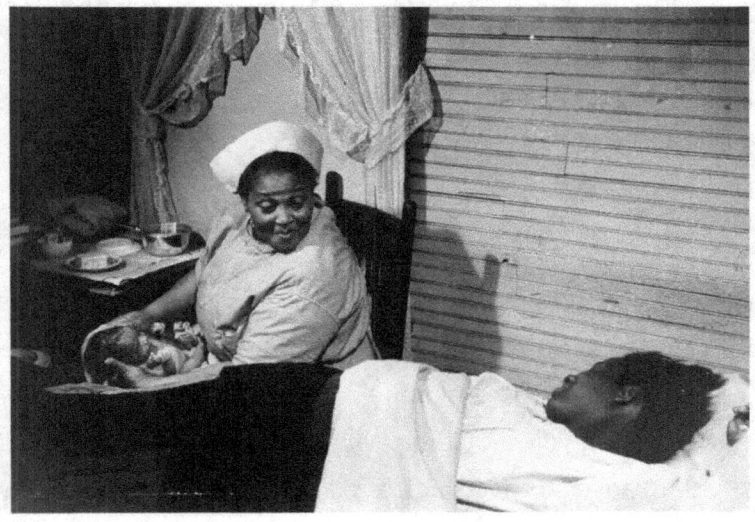

Figure 11-1. Doulas have always been a traditional fixture in the African American birthing experience.

5. Never check into a hospital alone.

It doesn't matter whether you're a queen or a rock star; always have a family member or trusted friend accompany you for the delivery. You'll receive better care and have a more satisfying birthing experience. This might sound like a piece of strange advice, but it's one borne out of personal observation at many fine hospitals over several decades. Doctors and nurses are human and respond differently, often more responsibly, when they realize they'll likely be held accountable by a third party witnessing the care. In addition, being in the throes of labor pain, you'll not be able to speak up and advocate for yourself. Well ahead of the due date, discuss your wants, choices, and preferences with your partner, friend, or family member so they can advocate on your behalf and speak up when there are any concerns.

6. An epidural is the best option for most women.

If you choose to have some form of pain control, the epidural is probably the best option. In the hands of competent anesthesia providers, the risks are minimal, and the benefits are significant. However, you should be aware of several short-term and long-term adverse effects before making your decision. Review the preceding chapters and keep in mind that some long-term adverse effects on the newborn, such as autism, ADHD, and lack of bonding, are only now being recognized. Therefore, the choice of epidural must be considered only after carefully reflecting on these potential adverse effects. Beyond your third pregnancy, an epidural is probably not the safest option for most women. We have discussed epidurals and their risks in the preceding chapters.

7. Labor pain gets less intense with each subsequent pregnancy.

The first pregnancy and first labor are often the most painful. After the fifth child, the labor pain is quite tolerable, and most women forego any spinal intervention.

8. Oxytocin will increase pain.

If your obstetrician is planning to use oxytocin to move labor along, ask for pain relief before starting the infusion. Oxytocin will produce strong, sustained contractions of the uterus, which will significantly increase the pain. The pain can be substantially reduced by having an epidural or spinal before the infusion. However, several studies point to a correlation between the maternal infusion of oxytocin and the occurrence of autism in children.

9. Some spines are not well suited for epidurals or spinals.

When giving an epidural or spinal for labor pain relief, the anesthesiologist must blindly—that is, without the use of X-rays—place the needle tip in the epidural space within the spine, which is only about 1 to 2 millimeters (about 0.08 inch) in width, located 8 to 10 centimeters deep below the skin, and exists in a gap between two adjacent vertebrae. It can be difficult to place an epidural in some circumstances. For example, if you are obese, have edema from toxemia of pregnancy, suffer from scoliosis or kyphosis of the spine, or have had prior spine surgery, it becomes challenging to place the epidural or spinal catheter properly. Under these circumstances, it's better to ask for an epidural or spinal early in your first stage of labor. Waiting until you're further along in your active phase of labor might make it difficult for you to sit or lie still without moving as the anesthesiologist struggles to place the catheter. The catheter can be placed when you're still comfortable during early labor and medications can be given later when your labor has adequately progressed.

10. Don't wait too long to ask for an epidural.

If you have decided on an epidural as your preferred mode of labor analgesia, ask for it earlier in your labor rather than later. Labor pain gets more intense as labor progresses. The ideal time to get an epidural is when the contractions are strong and regular and the cervix is dilated about 3 to 4 centimeters. If you wait too long, say 7 to 8 centimeters, then the fetal head will be farther down in the pelvis, pushing up against the perineal floor, making it difficult for you to sit still for the procedure. Experience shows complications from an epidural are significantly higher, and the block is often patchy, insufficient, unilateral, or of poor quality when performed in later stages of labor.

Keeping these ten best practices in mind during your pregnancy and being prepared to face the circumstances ahead increases your chance of having an enjoyable birthing experience.

Chapter 12

MAKING THE RIGHT CHOICE

I have outlined in this book most of the currently available techniques for pain relief during labor. Think and reflect on these options. Discuss your feelings with your physician, partner, friends, and family. No one method is superior to another. All of them pose varying amounts of risks to you and the baby while offering different magnitudes of pain relief. Candidly evaluate your level of pain tolerance. Has your pregnancy been normal? Have you given birth before this pregnancy? What is your overall philosophical attitude toward life and medical interventions? Hopefully, your final choice will be safe for you and the baby and consistent with your values.

As we saw in the data outlined in previous chapters, not every woman in labor needs an epidural. If you are fit and do not suffer from any pregnancy-related complications, you probably do not need an epidural. If you have reasonable pain tolerance and support of good family or friends, then irrespective of your parity, you are better off without an epidural. The risks associated with an epidural outweigh the benefits if you have already given birth to two or more children. The risks are also not in your favor if you or your partner is 35 years of age or older or has a family history of autism spectrum disorder.

You may wonder as to what you gain from foregoing an epidural. There are many benefits to the mother and child from avoiding an epidural. You save yourself and the child from a plethora of immediate, short-term, and lifelong complications. The immediate potential complications include injuries to your spinal nerves, spinal headache, low blood pressure, slow heart rate, inability to breathe, fetal distress, total spinal, and death.

Remember, the epidural complications are like the Russian Matryoshka dolls; more and more complications are often nestled within each intervention aimed at correcting these complications. Because the epidural blocks the sensations from your uterus and relaxes your abdominal and pelvic muscles, you will probably need an oxytocin infusion. Oxytocin itself has several side effects, including increasing the intensity of your pain, risk of uterine rupture, low blood pressure, nausea, and vomiting. It is also known to cause harm to your baby, particularly if the baby happens to be male.

Epidural also increases your chances of cesarean section, often due to failure of labor to progress. Cesarean sections have their own set of complications, including infection, bleeding, and injury to your bladder, ureters, and bowels. In the long term, you may develop adhesions in your abdomen, leading to bowel obstruction, ureteral obstruction, or chronic abdominal pain.

Epidural also increases your chances of instrumental delivery. Because you cannot push effectively, your obstetrician will have to pull the baby out with forceps or a vacuum extractor. Both can cause significant injury to the brain and face of the child. This includes facial bones or skull fractures, intracranial bleeding, or injury to the cervical spine. Soft tissue organs such as the ears, nose, and eyes could also be crushed or bruised. All of these injuries could contribute to cerebral palsy or other developmental disorders in the child. The injuries to the mother's birth canal are also significant with instrumental delivery.

Most often, the application of forceps will require an episiotomy, which could get infected, causing chronic pelvic pain, sinuses, fistulae, or distortion of the vaginal outlet. The forceps can also damage the pelvic floor, leading to future urinary incontinence or fecal incontinence. In the long term, the epidural causes more harm to the child than the mother.

Traumatic birth as a result of instrumental delivery or delayed cesarean section in the presence of fetal distress is a significant cause of cerebral palsy in the child. Now there are convincing studies that show an increased occurrence of autism and autism spectrum disorders in women who undergo epidural analgesia. Since oxytocin is often used to counter the paralytic effects of epidural and hence one has to look at the adverse effects of oxytocin as well. Synthetic oxytocin, administered as an intravenous infusion, adversely impacts the intrinsic natural oxytocin in both the mother and child. Studies now show increased autism and autism spectrum disorders in women who receive oxytocin infusion. The children born to these mothers may also lack family bonding, exhibit antisocial behaviors, and suffer mental illness. Many of these adverse effects may not be evident or diagnosed until much later in the child's development or entry into school. When these delayed complications are discovered, the triggering event, the epidural, will be a distant forgotten memory.

Despite the myriads of potential complications, the epidural is an effective and predictable mode of pain relief. In women who have low pain tolerance and are having their first or second baby, the epidural is an excellent choice. In certain expecting mothers with pregnancy-related ailments, such as gestational diabetes, hypertension, or preeclampsia, the epidural may have therapeutic benefits in addition to providing pain relief. The epidural may also provide therapeutic benefit to a small segment of women who should avoid excessive straining in labor; these include those with congestive heart failure, those with asthma, those who suffer from pulmonary hypertension, certain forms of congenital heart disease, morbid obesity, and those with history of intracranial bleeding or retinal detachment.

We are left with a group of women in the middle, who would rather not have an epidural but still need some form of pain relief to temper the harshness of contractions. For this group, intravenous pain medications are a good choice. These include opioids, dexmedetomidine, and ketamine. Nitrous oxide inhalation is also a reasonable choice. In women who need more, regional blocks such as paracervical block, pudendal nerve block, or even single-shot spinal or a caudal block may be appropriate.

For women with high pain tolerance or who have had multiple children in the past, natural childbirth or the adoption of alternative medical interventions might be the best choice. These interventions are often downplayed in modern obstetrical practice because there is very little financial incentive to advocate for them. Also, there is very little research on them due to a lack of interest from physician organizations. Yet, some of these measures are very effective in mitigating pain and distress while lacking the serious complications of an epidural. Dulas, for example, make an enormous difference in the outcome and experience of childbirth, irrespective of the mother's parity. If you can pay for them, I strongly recommend employing their services. Water birth, hypnosis, acupressure, yoga, TENS, massage, and meditation all provide incremental benefits to the receptive mind. The great advantage of these holistic interventions is that you can try them, and if they are ineffective and the pain is beyond your tolerance, you can always ask for and receive an epidural. You never foreclose more invasive interventions simply because you give less invasive measures a chance to work.

Ultimately, you should choose a pain relief option that is consistent with your values and safe for you and the baby. In defining your values, you must consider what you are willing to sacrifice now for the long-term benefits of you and your child. On a practical level, honestly consider your pain tolerance, how strong your support system is, your faith in God, and the resources available at your healthcare facility. I hope the information I have provided in this book will help you make the right choice.

I wish you and your baby a happy, healthy, and joyous birthing experience.

APPENDIX I.
PACKING HOSPITAL BAGS

In the month leading up to your expected delivery date, it is crucial that you pack all your necessities and have them ready to grab when labor begins. I have seen too many women arrive at the emergency department without any belongings and exclaim, "My water broke!" They walk in empty-handed, expecting the hospital to take care of both them and their baby for the next three to four days. While hospitals do their best to accommodate patients, this scenario often results in an uncomfortable experience for everyone involved.

You must pack three duffel bags that are easily accessible when labor starts (see Figure AI-1). One bag should be for you, one for your partner, and one for the baby. Additionally, ensure that you have an infant car seat prepared well before your hospital stay (see Figure AI-2).

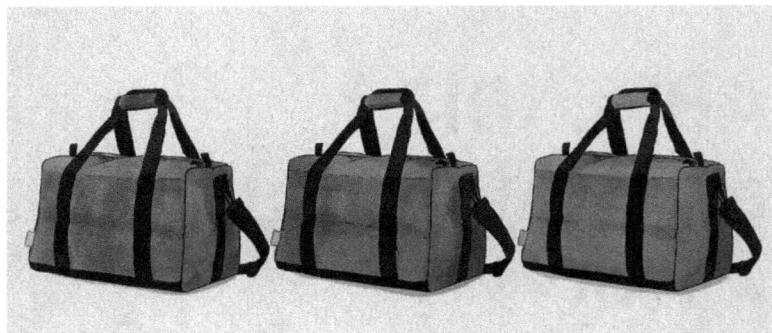

Figure AI-1. Pack your bags in advance for the trip to the hospital on the expected date. Pack separate bags for you, your partner, and the baby.

Taking the time to carefully plan and pack these items will significantly enhance your hospital experience and prevent you from forgetting anything important. Being well-prepared will give you greater control over what takes place in the following days. Use the checklist provided to verify you have all the essential items packed and ready to go.

Your Bag

   1. Hospital paperwork, ID, and insurance card

   2. Birth plan

   3. Socks

   4. Slippers

   5. Bathrobe, underwear, bras

6. Nightgowns, loose-fitting clothes

7. Heavy-duty maternity pads

8. Toothpaste, toothbrush, deodorant, hairbrush, and other toiletries

9. Body lotion, massage oil, and lip balm

10. Comfortable pillows

11. Light entertainment: music, DVDs, tablets, laptops, or books

12. Eye masks, noise-canceling earphones

13. Glasses or contact lenses

14. Cell phone and charger

15. Snacks, high-protein drinks, and water

Your Partner's Bag

1. Phone, camera, video camera, chargers

2. Snacks, soft drinks, water

3. Light entertainment: music, DVDs, tablets, laptops, or books

4. Toiletries

5. Pillows and small blankets

6. Credit cards, some cash

7. A few small garbage bags

Your Baby's Bag

1. Bodysuits

2. Socks and mittens

3. Hats

4. Diapers

5. Baby wipes

6. Diaper rash cream

7. Soft baby towels

8. Baby wraps

9. Pacifiers

10. Diaper changing mat

11. Round-tipped nail scissors

In addition to these three bags, ensure you have an **infant car seat** ready to take to the hospital.

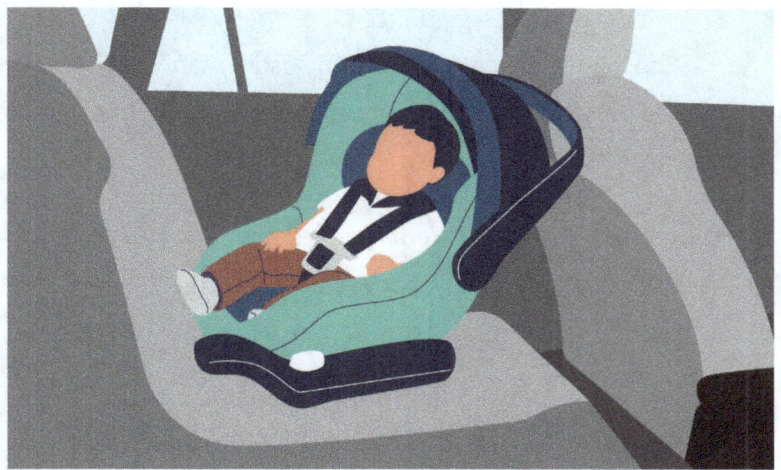

Figure AI-2. The baby should always be properly secured in an infant car seat while riding in an automobile.

Setting up the infant seat is a three-step process:

1. Ensure the infant seat is assembled correctly. Some can be detachable and hand-carried, while others convert to a stroller. Make sure you follow the manufacturer's instructions.

2. Ensure you know how to anchor the infant seat to the car seat safely. Some seats have an easy latch system that clips the infant seat to the car seat. In others, you must use the car's seat belt to anchor the infant seat.

3. You should know how to snuggly secure the infant to the infant seat. Infant seat belts should be neither too tight nor too loose. You should be able to freely insert your fingers between the seat belt and the baby's chest. Many fire departments, hospitals, and police depart-

ments offer free guidance on properly securing and using infant car seats. Improperly used infant car seats can be very dangerous. If in doubt, seek the help of these professionals.

Being prepared with these items packed and ready will give you peace of mind, assuring you that you haven't forgotten anything essential. It will be a good, positive start to your birthing experience.

APPENDIX II. COMPREHENSIVE BIRTH PLAN

This appendix will help you craft your birth plan. A birth plan communicates your preferences for labor and delivery. Not only does it convey your wishes to the medical staff, but it also serves as a tool to prepare for the birth event. Creating a birth plan encourages you to consider various aspects of labor and delivery. This reflective endeavor helps you feel more prepared as you approach the delivery date.

Start by discussing your thoughts and concerns with your obstetrician. They can provide valuable insights into what is feasible and what interventions are mandatory standards of care to maintain the safety and well-being of the baby and yourself. Then, deliberate on your preferences and what is feasible with your partner, family, and friends (see Figure AII-1).

Afterward, using the template provided in this appendix, draft your birth plan. The birth plan must be realistic, feasible given your individual circumstances, and consistent with your values. The plan must also have sufficient specific instructions in situations where you cannot voice your preferences due to pain or other complications. Under these circumstances, the plan will act as your advocate, guiding the medical staff to perform in alignment with your wishes and preferences. You should share a copy of the birth plan with the hospital staff at the time of admission for delivery, or preferably several days ahead of time. In most hospitals, your birth plan will become part of your medical record.

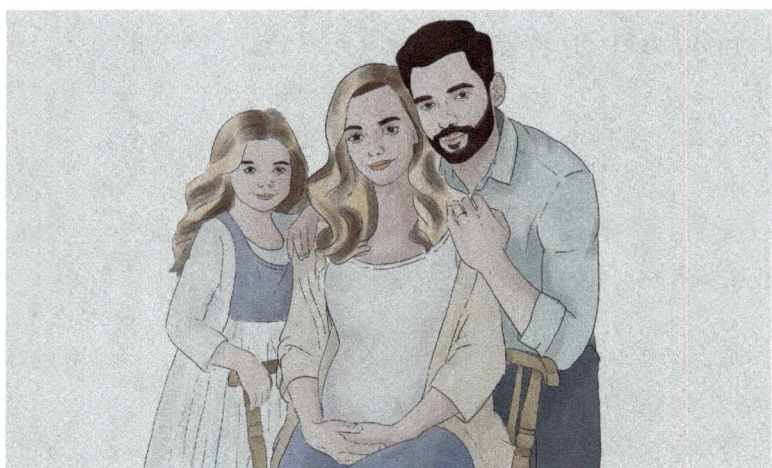

Figure AII-1. Create a sensible birth plan in consultation with your physician, partner, family, and friends. A well-crafted birth plan will allow events to unfold in an orderly and safe manner.

BIRTH PLAN

Preamble: This birth plan outlines my preferences for labor and delivery. I trust my healthcare providers to use their professional judgment and expertise to ensure the safety and well-being of my baby and myself. If there is a choice in the matter, this document contains my preferences. I understand that clinical circumstances may necessitate deviations from this plan. I rely on my healthcare providers to make informed decisions based on the best available medical evidence and to prioritize the health and safety of my baby and myself.

I. Personal Information

NAME

_____

DATE OF BIRTH

_____

TELEPHONE

_____

EMAIL

_____

ADDRESS

_____

_____

_____

II. Birth Partner/Spouse

NAME

_____

DATE OF BIRTH

_____

TELEPHONE

_____

EMAIL

_____

ADDRESS

_____

_____

_____

III. Baby Due Date

_____

IV. Baby's Name

_____

☐   To be decided later

V. Hospital/Birthing Center Information

NAME OF FACILITY

_____

ADDRESS

_____

_____

_____

_____

TELEPHONE

_____

VI. Hospital/Birthing Center Information

	NAME	TELEPHONE

OBSTETRICIAN

_____

MIDWIFE

_____

DOULA

_____

PEDIATRICIAN

_____

ANESTHESIOLOGIST

_____

NURSE

_____

VII. Medical History

HEIGHT

_____

WEIGHT

_____

No. PRIOR
PREGNANCIES

_____

No. PRIOR
BIRTHING

_____

DIFFICULTIES WITH PRIOR PREGNANCY   Yes ☐   No ☐

PRIOR CESAREAN SECTIONS   Yes ☐   No ☐

PRIOR FORCEPS DELIVERIES   Yes ☐   No ☐

PRIOR SURGERIES, IF ANY

_____

_____

ALLERGIES

_____

SMOKING HISTORY

_____

ALCOHOL USE

_____

RECREATIONAL DRUGS Yes ☐ No ☐

DIABETES Yes ☐ No ☐

HYPERTENSION Yes ☐ No ☐

ASTHMA Yes ☐ No ☐

BLEEDING DISORDER Yes ☐ No ☐

OTHER ILLNESS

_____

Current Prescription Medications

☐ Pain Medications

_____

☐ Antidepressants

_____

☐ Blood Pressure
   Medications

_____

☐ Asthma Inhalers

_____

☐ Diabetic Medications

_____

☐ Insulin Injections

_____

☐ Other Medicines

_____

VIII. During Labor

My Preference During Early Labor Contractions:

☐ Walking with assistance

_____

☐ Lying down with the
head of the bed raised

_____

☐ Lying down on my side
with my head raised

_____

☐ Standing up with
assistance

_____

☐ Sitting in a warm
bathtub

_____

☐ Doula assistance

_____

☐ Sitting up in a birthing
stool

_____

☐ Sitting on a birthing ball

_____

☐ Other

_____

I Prefer the Delivery Room to Be:

☐ Quiet room   ☐ Lights dimmed   ☐ Television off

☐ Background music   ☐ Extra pillows   ☐ Nothing special

I Prefer the Following Visitors:

☐ No visitors

_____

☐ Spouse/partner

_____

- ☐ Parents/siblings/children

  _____

- ☐ Relatives

  _____

- ☐ Friends

  _____

- ☐ Adoption parents

  _____

- ☐ Pastor/spiritual
  counselor

  _____

- ☐ Doula

  _____

- ☐ Other

  _____

My Preference for Labor Pain Management:

- ☐ I leave it to the discretion of my obstetrician

  _____

- ☐ I leave it to the discretion of my
  anesthesiologist

  _____

- ☐ Epidural – single shot or continuous

  _____

- ☐ Spinal – single shot or continuous

  _____

- ☐ Paracervical block

  _____

- ☐ Pudendal nerve block

  _____

- ☐ Other forms of nerve blocks

  _____

- ☐ Oral pain medications

  _____

- [ ] Intravenous pain medications, including opioids

    _____

- [ ] Nitrous oxide–oxygen breathing mixture

    _____

- [ ] Doula-assisted continuous support

    _____

- [ ] Massage therapy

    _____

- [ ] Deep breathing and positive visualization

    _____

- [ ] Acupuncture and acupressure

    _____

- [ ] Allow natural response to pain – squeezing/shaking/primal screaming

    _____

- [ ] Therapist-induced hypnosis

    _____

- [ ] Other

    _____

- [ ] Epidural – if trial of other forms of pain relief fails, and it is safe to do so

    _____

My Preference for Cervical Ripening:

Foley catheter   Yes [ ]   No [ ]

Misoprostol (Cytotec®)   Yes [ ]   No [ ]

- [ ] I leave it to the discretion of my obstetrician.

My Preference for Induction of Labor:

- [ ] I do not want to hasten my labor through the infusion of oxytocin (Pitocin).

- [ ] I leave the use of oxytocin to the discretion of my obstetrician.

- [ ] I prefer to avoid artificial rupture of membranes (AROM).

- [ ] I leave the decision on AROM to the discretion of my obstetrician.

IX. During Delivery

My Positioning Preference During Delivery:

- ☐ Standing up with assistance
- ☐ Squatting
- ☐ Semi-reclined with my legs up (lithotomy position)
- ☐ Semi-recumbent in the water tub
- ☐ As considered appropriate by my obstetrician

I Prefer the Following Individuals In the Delivery Room With Me:

- ☐ No family members or friends. Only the healthcare providers.

My spouse/partner	Yes ☐	No ☐
My mother/father	Yes ☐	No ☐
My siblings	Yes ☐	No ☐
My friends	Yes ☐	No ☐

Names of friends: _____

My other children   Yes ☐   No ☐

Other individuals (example: spiritual counselor, pastor, adoption mother, legal representative)   Yes ☐   No ☐

Names of others: _____

My Preference for an Episiotomy:

- ☐ Okay to perform "routine" prophylactic episiotomy
- ☐ Only as a last resort to avoid a significant perineal tear
- ☐ Leave it to the discretion of my obstetrician
- ☐ No episiotomy, even at the risk of perineal tear

My Preference for the Use of Forceps to Aid In Delivery:

- ☐ Do not use forceps or a vacuum extractor
- ☐ Use forceps or a vacuum extractor only as a last resort
- ☐ Leave it to the discretion of my obstetrician

In the Case of a Cesarean Delivery, My Choice of Anesthesia:

- ☐ I prefer to be asleep under general anesthesia.
- ☐ I prefer to be awake under spinal or epidural anesthesia.
- ☐ I leave it to the discretion of my anesthesiologist and obstetrician.

In the Case of a Cesarean Delivery, I Prefer the Following Individual to Be Present With Me In the Operating Room:

- ☐ My spouse/partner
- ☐ My sister/mother
- ☐ My friend
- ☐ Other name: _____

Photography of Birth:

- ☐ I do not want a picture or video of the baby.
- ☐ I want a picture or video of the baby immediately after delivery.
- ☐ I want a picture or video of the baby and me.
- ☐ I want a picture or video of the baby with my spouse/partner.

IX. During Delivery

Resuscitation of the Baby After Birth:

- ☐ I prefer delayed cord clamping for at least 2-3 minutes.
- ☐ I prefer no routine eye drops, vitamin K, or Hep B vaccine without consent.
- ☐ I prefer a pediatrician or family physician to resuscitate my baby.
- ☐ I leave the baby's resuscitation to the discretion of my obstetrician.

Immediately After the Birth of My Bab, I Prefer the Following Bonding Rituals:

Holding my baby skin-to-skin for several minutes ☐ Yes ☐ No

Keep my baby by my side or on my chest for a few hours ☐ Yes ☐ No

I prefer bathing, foot printing, length measurement, and weighing to be delayed until I have spent sufficient skin-to-skin time with the baby ☐ Yes ☐ No

My Preference for Feeding the Baby:

☐ I prefer to breastfeed the baby.

☐ I prefer to formula-feed the baby.

☐ I prefer to breastfeed with consultation from a lactation consultant.

My Preference for Keeping the Baby In the Nursery:

☐ I always prefer to keep the baby in my room.

☐ I prefer to keep the baby in my room only during the day.

☐ I prefer to keep the baby in my room only during feeding.

My Preference for Circumcision If the Baby Is Male:

☐ No circumcision

☐ Circumcision under local anesthesia before discharge from the hospital

☐ Circumcision at a later date

Other Instructions / Notes

I affirm under penalty of perjury that this birth plan accurately represents my wishes for the labor and delivery of my baby.

_____   _____

Patient Signature   Date

APPENDIX III. THE LANGUAGE OF OBSTETRICS

If you are unfamiliar with the medical field, it will be beneficial to understand the essential obstetrical terminology physicians and nurses use in their practice. This will help you better understand your obstetrician and effectively articulate your wants:

Gravid means pregnant. **Gravida** is the total number of pregnancies a woman has experienced, regardless of the outcome.

Parity means births. This could mean full-term birth, preterm birth, or abortion. When your obstetrician speaks of G2P1, for example, she means the woman is pregnant for the second time and has given birth to one infant or aborted once in the past.

A **parturient** is a woman in labor who is about to give birth or has recently given birth.

An **infant** is a live-born baby from birth until one year of life.

A **term infant** is born between 37 and 40 weeks of gestation.

A **preterm infant** is born between 20 and 37 weeks of gestation. Preterm infants need to be at least 500 grams in weight to survive.

A **post-term infant** is a baby born after 42 weeks of gestation.

A **neonate** is a newborn baby up until 28 days of life.

A **fetus** refers to an unborn child from the time of an embryo to birth. This includes the period of growth from nine weeks following fertilization to the time of birth.

Fetal heart tones are sounds created by the beating heart of the fetus and are detectable by Doppler after 10 weeks of gestation. A regular fetal heart rate is 110 to 160 beats per minute.

The **cervix** is the muscular ring at the lower end of the uterus, which remains closed until the onset of labor. The cervix opens into the vagina. It's about three to four centimeters long and has an internal and external opening; as the head of the fetus descends, the internal opening dilates first, followed gradually by the dilation of the external opening. These two processes are called cervical effacement and cervical dilation. When the cervix is fully effaced and dilated, the external opening is 10 centimeters or greater in diameter.

Braxton-Hicks contractions are less painful contractions of the uterus occurring in the final four to eight weeks of pregnancy. They are often irregular and may slowly increase in frequency, lasting several hours. They are the common cause of "false labor." They are distinguished from actual labor by the lack of cervical changes in response to the contractions.

The **station of fetal head** is the extent of the fetal head's descent into the pelvis in relation to the ischial spines of the pelvis (see Figure AIII-1). Station zero refers to the leading edge of the fetal head in line with the interspinous line. A measurement of +2 denotes 2 cm below the interspinous line, and –2 denotes 2 cm above the interspinous line.

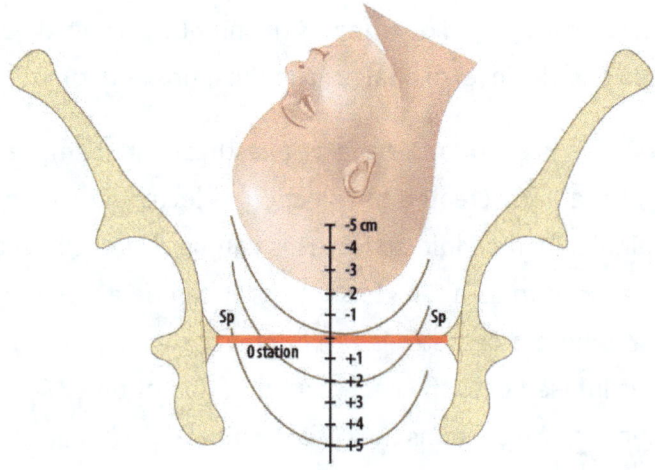

Figure AIII-1. The fetal head is at -2 station. At station 0, the head is fully engaged within the pelvis.

An **epidural** is a state of analgesia or anesthesia affecting certain parts of the body created by injection of local anesthetic into the spinal epidural space. The local anesthetic prevents the spinal nerve impulses from reaching the spinal cord and ultimately the brain. When lower concentrations of local anesthetic agents are used, predominantly the sensory impulses are blocked, and the motor impulses are relatively spared. This state is referred to as **epidural analgesia**.

When higher concentrations of local anesthetic agents are used, both sensory and motor nerve impulses are blocked. This state is referred to as **epidural anesthesia**. An epidural analgesia can be easily converted to an epidural anesthesia by injecting higher concentrations of local anesthetics. During labor, an epidural analgesia is often performed in the upper lumbar spine, providing pain relief from uterine contractions. The volume of local anesthetic injected determines the number of spinal nerves blocked and the level of analgesia in the limbs and torso.

A **spinal** is a state of analgesia or anesthesia affecting certain parts of the body created by injection of local anesthetic into the spinal subarachnoid space. This can be a single injection, often referred to as a "single shot," or it can be a "continuous spinal," where a catheter is left in place, and the local anesthetic is infused over the necessary duration of time. The subarachnoid space contains the cerebrospinal fluid (CSF), and the local anesthetic mixes with the CSF and acts directly on the spinal cord and spinal nerve roots. Lower concentrations of local anesthetics will predominantly block the sensory impulses, and higher concentrations of local anesthetics will block both sensory and motor nerve impulses. The level of the spinal block will depend on the baricity (relative density) of the local anesthetic preparation in relation to the CSF. If the spinal is performed with the parturient sitting up, and the local anesthetic preparation is hyperbaric (denser than CSF), the local anesthetic will sink to lower levels of the spine and cause analgesia or anesthesia of sacral and lower lumbar spinal segments. This is often referred to as caudal analgesia. The level of spinal analgesia or anesthesia will depend on the baricity of the local anesthetic preparation and the position of the spine immediately following the injection.

A **bolus** is a large dose of medication, either by volume, concentration, or weight, administered to a patient in the form of an injection. It is in contrast to administering smaller incremental doses of the same medication in the form of an infusion. Local anesthetics are often bolused at the beginning of an epidural infusion. Intravenous fluids can also be bolused to improve a falling blood pressure.

An **episiotomy** is a surgical incision made in the perineum and vagina to enlarge the vaginal outlet. It is performed in the region between the vaginal outlet and the anus. It can be in the midline or mediolateral, extending to the sides. An episiotomy makes it easier to deliver a large head or other malpresentations of the fetus. It also permits the easy application of forceps. It is repaired after the delivery of the fetus and placenta.

Pitocin is the brand name for the synthetic version of the naturally occurring hormone **oxytocin**. Oxytocin (Pitocin) causes strong contraction of the uterus and helps in expelling the fetus and placenta during labor. Oxytocin also causes the ejection of milk during breastfeeding. Oxytocin may also possess other neuropsychological effects, such as mother-infant bonding.

Naturally produced oxytocin may have different central nervous system effects than peripherally administered synthetic oxytocin.

There are three **stages of labor**:

- First Stage: Interval between the onset of labor pains and full cervical dilatation.

- Second Stage: Interval between the full cervical dilatation and delivery of the infant.

- Third Stage: Interval between the delivery of the infant and the delivery of the placenta.

Pregnancy is divided into three **trimesters** of approximately 12 to 14 weeks (about three months) each. The first trimester lasts from conception to the end of week 12, the second trimester lasts from week 13 to week 26, and the third trimester lasts from week 27 to the birth of the baby (week 40).

A **vaginal examination** is the inspection and palpation of the female genitalia (see Figure AIII-2). It is often referred to as a pelvic examination. In obstetrics, it is used to assess the ripening, dilatation, and effacement of the uterine cervix. It can be used to determine the descent and station of the fetal head. It is also used to diagnose abnormal bleeding, tumors, pelvic pain, and sexually transmitted infections.

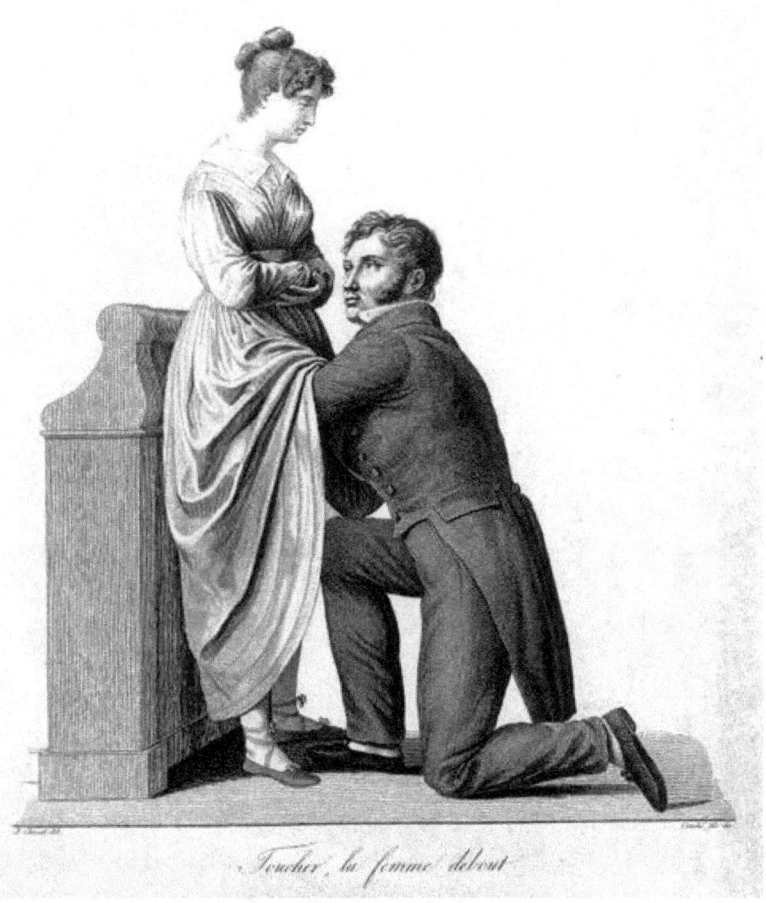

Figure AIII-2. Illustration of how to perform a modest vaginal examination.

REFERENCES

1. Taffel, S.M., P.J. Placek, and T. Liss, *Trends in the United States cesarean section rate and reasons for the 1980-85 rise.* Am J Public Health, 1987. 77(8): p. 955-9.

2. CDC, *Births: Final Data for 2022.* 2024, https://dx.doi.or g/10.15620/cdc:145588: Hyattsville, MD.

3. Harkins, J., et al., *Survey of the Factors Associated with a Woman's Choice to Have an Epidural for Labor Analgesia.* Anesthesiol Res Pract, 2010.

4. Seijmonsbergen-Schermers, A.E., et al., *Variations in use of childbirth interventions in 13 high-income countries: A multinational cross-sectional study.* PLoS Med, 2020. 17(5): p. e1003103.

5. Mikulinsky, O. *When Childbirth Cost $100.* 2023; Available from: https://www.cryo-cell.com/blog/april-2017 /when-childbirth-cost-100-dollars.

6. Rivelli, E. *How Much Does It Cost To Have A Baby? 2024 Averages.* 2024; Available from:

https://www.forbes.com/advisor/health-insurance/ave
rage-childbirth-cost/#:~:text=Giving%20birth%20costs
%20%2418%2C865%20on,(KFF)%20Health%20Syste
m%20Tracker.

7. Fox, H., et al., *A cascade of interventions: A classification tree analysis of the determinants of primary cesareans in Australian public hospitals.* Birth, 2021. 48(2): p. 209-220.

8. Lothian, J.A., *Healthy Birth Practice #4: Avoid Interventions Unless They Are Medically Necessary.* J Perinat Educ, (4): p. 198-206.

9. Fernández-Arroyo, M.F., *Childbirth education: comparative analysis*, in *Childbirth*. 2019, IntechOpen.

10. Lederman, R.P., et al., *Preparation for Labor.* Psychosocial Adaptation to Pregnancy: Seven Dimensions of Maternal Development, 2020: p. 165-197.

11. Ramalingam, G.D., S. Gayatri, and J.P. Amirtham, *Challenges Facing during Pregnancy and Measures to Overcome.* Global Women's Health, 2021: p. 1-16.

12. Kannan, S., R.N. Jamison, and S. Datta, *Maternal satisfaction and pain control in women electing natural childbirth.* Reg Anesth Pain Med, 2001. 26(5): p. 468-72.

13. Ros, A., et al., *Epidural anaesthesia for labour: does it influence the mode of delivery?* Arch Gynecol Obstet, 2007. 275(4): p. 269-74.

14. Ballesteros-Meseguer, C., et al., *Episiotomy and its relationship to various clinical variables that influence its performance.* Rev Lat Am Enfermagem, 2016. 24: p. e2793.

15. Clesse, C., et al., *Episiotomy practices in France: epidemiology and risk factors in non-operative vaginal deliveries.* Sci Rep, 2020. 10(1): p. 20208.

16. Loewenberg-Weisband, Y., et al., *Epidural analgesia and severe perineal tears: a literature review and large cohort study.* J Matern Fetal Neonatal Med, 2014. 27(18): p. 1864-9.

17. Gregory, S.G., et al., *Association of autism with induced or augmented childbirth in North Carolina Birth Record (1990-1998) and Education Research (1997-2007) databases.* JAMA Pediatr, 2013. 167(10): p. 959-66.

18. Hanley, G.E., et al., *Association of Epidural Analgesia During Labor and Delivery With Autism Spectrum Disorder in Offspring.* JAMA, 2021. 326(12): p. 1178-1185.

19. Mikkelsen, A.P., et al., *Association of Labor Epidural Analgesia With Autism Spectrum Disorder in Children.* JAMA, 2021. 326(12): p. 1170-1177.

20. Wall-Wieler, E., et al., *Association of Epidural Labor Analgesia With Offspring Risk of Autism Spectrum Disorders.* JAMA Pediatrics, 2021. 175(7): p. 698-705.

21. Wong, C.A. and H. Stevens, *Labor Epidural Analgesia*

and Autism Spectrum Disorder: Is There an Association? JAMA, 2021. 326(12): p. 1155-1157.

22. Qiu, C., et al., *Association of Labor Epidural Analgesia, Oxytocin Exposure, and Risk of Autism Spectrum Disorders in Children.* JAMA Netw Open, 2023. 6(7): p. e2324630.

23. Qiu, C., et al., *Association Between Epidural Analgesia During Labor and Risk of Autism Spectrum Disorders in Offspring.* JAMA Pediatr, 2020. 174(12): p. 1168-1175.

24. Murphy, M.S.Q., et al., *Exposure to Intrapartum Epidural Analgesia and Risk of Autism Spectrum Disorder in Offspring.* JAMA Netw Open, 2022. 5(5): p. e2214273.

25. Golub, M.S. and S.L. Germann, *Perinatal bupivacaine and infant behavior in rhesus monkeys.* Neurotoxicol Teratol, 1998. 20(1): p. 29-41.

26. Qiu, C., et al., *Association of Labor Epidural Analgesia, Oxytocin Exposure, and Risk of Autism Spectrum Disorders in Children.* JAMA Network Open, 2023. 6(7): p. e2324630-e2324630.

27. Hotoft, D. and R.D. Maimburg, *Epidural analgesia during birth and adverse neonatal outcomes: A population-based cohort study.* Women Birth, 2021. 34(3): p. e286-e291.

28. Costley, P.L. and C.E. East, *Oxytocin augmentation of labour in women with epidural analgesia for reducing*

operative deliveries. Cochrane Database Syst Rev, 2013. (7): p. CD009241.

29. Weisman, O., et al., *The association between 2D:4D ratio and cognitive empathy is contingent on a common polymorphism in the oxytocin receptor gene (OXTR rs53576).* Psychoneuroendocrinology, 2015. 58: p. 23-32.

30. Weisman, O., et al., *Oxytocin-augmented labor and risk for autism in males.* Behav Brain Res, 2015. 284: p. 207-12.

31. Feldman, R., et al., *Evidence for a neuroendocrinological foundation of human affiliation: plasma oxytocin levels across pregnancy and the postpartum period predict mother-infant bonding.* Psychol Sci, 2007. 18(11): p. 965-70.

32. Levine, A., et al., *Oxytocin during pregnancy and early postpartum: individual patterns and maternal-fetal attachment.* Peptides, 2007. 28(6): p. 1162-9.

33. Rahm, V.A., et al., *Plasma oxytocin levels in women during labor with or without epidural analgesia: a prospective study.* Acta Obstet Gynecol Scand, 2002. 81(11): p. 1033-9.

34. Buckley, S., et al., *Maternal and newborn plasma oxytocin levels in response to maternal synthetic oxytocin administration during labour, birth and postpartum - a systematic review with implications for the function*

of the oxytocinergic system. BMC Pregnancy Childbirth, 2023. 23(1): p. 137.

35. Rooks, J.P., *Oxytocin as a "high alert medication": a multilayered challenge to the status quo.* Birth, 2009. 36(4): p. 345-8.

36. Joel, S., et al., *Low-dose ketamine infusion for labor analgesia: A double-blind, randomized, placebo controlled clinical trial.* Saudi J Anaesth, 2014. 8(1): p. 6-10.

37. Delavari, A., M. Dehgan, and M. Lak, *Evaluating the Effect of Dexmedetomidine Intravenous Infusion on Labour Pain Management in Primipara Pregnant Women: A Nonrandomised Clinical Trial Study.* Rom J Anaesth Intensive Care, 2021. 28(1): p. 10-18.

38. Nodine, P.M., et al., *Nitrous Oxide Use During Labor: Satisfaction, Adverse Effects, and Predictors of Conversion to Neuraxial Analgesia.* J Midwifery Womens Health, 2020. 65(3): p. 335-341.

39. Rimsza, R.R., et al., *Time from neuraxial anesthesia placement to delivery is inversely proportional to umbilical arterial cord pH at scheduled cesarean delivery.* Am J Obstet Gynecol, 2019. 220(4): p. 389 e1-389 e9.

40. Zewdu, D., et al., *Exploring factors influencing skin incision to the delivery time and their impact on neonatal outcomes among emergency cesarean deliveries indicated for non-reassured fetal heart rate status.* Front

Pediatr, 2023. 11: p. 1224508.

41. Adams, J.B., et al., *Evidence based recommendations for an optimal prenatal supplement for women in the US: vitamins and related nutrients.* Matern Health Neonatol Perinatol, 2022. 8(1): p. 4.

42. Adams, J.B., et al., *Evidence-Based Recommendations for an Optimal Prenatal Supplement for Women in the U.S., Part Two: Minerals.* Nutrients, 2021. 13(6).

43. Corrigan, L., et al., *The characteristics and effectiveness of pregnancy yoga interventions: a systematic review and meta-analysis.* BMC Pregnancy Childbirth, 2022. 22(1): p. 250.

44. Smith, C.A., et al., *Acupuncture or acupressure for pain management during labour.* Cochrane Database Syst Rev, 2020. 2(2): p. CD009232.

45. Nwanodi, O.B., *Labor pain treated with acupuncture or acupressure.* Chinese Medicine, 2016. 7(4): p. 133-152.

46. Heap, M., *Hypnotherapy - A Handbook.* 2nd ed. 2012, Milton Keynes, UK: Open University Press.

47. Madden, K., et al., *Hypnosis for pain management during labour and childbirth.* Cochrane Database Syst Rev, 2016. (5): p. CD009356.

48. Sobczak, A., et al., *The Effect of Doulas on Maternal and Birth Outcomes: A Scoping Review.* Cureus, 2023. 15(5):

p. e39451.

49. Reschke, M.M., et al., *Choice of local anaesthetic for epidural caesarean section: a Bayesian network meta-analysis.* Anaesthesia, 2020. 75(5): p. 674-682.

FIGURE CREDITS

Figure 2-2. Ms. Jessica Ross, who lost her baby due to excessive traction from forceps, and her partner, at a news conference with their attorney. (Copyright 2023, Sudhin Thanawala / AP).

Figure 4-4. Sha Asia Semple's death from total spinal sparked protests across New York City. Many women were unaware of this complication from epidural. (Copyright 2020 Alamy Inc.)

Figure 7-2. Maternal mortality by race in the US (2022). [National Center for Health Statistics. 2023 DOI: https://dx.doi.org/10.15620/cdc:124678].

Figure 7-3. Infant mortality by race in the US (2022). [National Center for Health Statistics. 2023. DOI: https://dx.doi.org/10.15620/cdc:131356].

Figure 9-5. Self-reported pain scores of 2,471 Southeast Asian women during subsequent pregnancies (Dr. R Subramanian, MBBS, DGO & Dr. S Sundaram, MBBS, FRCS).

Figure 11.1. Smithsonian. National Museum of African American History and Culture.

Figure AIII-2. Illustration of how to perform a modest vaginal examination. Jacques-Pierre Maygrier's Atlas—Nouvelles Demonstrations d' Accouchements. Paris, France (1822). [Wellcome Collection. https://wellcomecollection.org/works/py2s64zh]

ABOUT THE AUTHOR

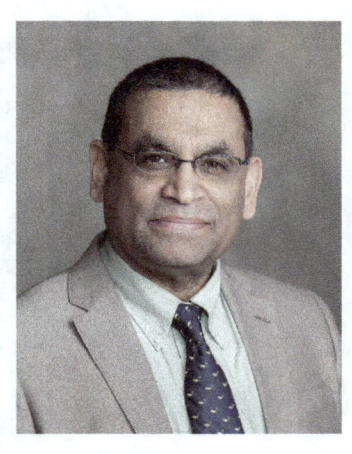

Dr. Matthew Kumar is a board-certified anesthesiologist and intensivist with over four decades of clinical experience. He combines practical expertise with deep compassion for managing pain during childbirth. Currently, he serves as the Chief of Anesthesiology Services at the Minneapolis VA Medical Center. Prior to this role, he practiced for more than 30 years as a Consultant in Anesthesiology and Critical Care Medicine at the Mayo Clinic in Rochester, Minnesota. Throughout his career, he has educated numerous medical students, nurses, residents, and graduate students. Dr. Kumar is also actively engaged in medical research and has participated in several clinical trials and holds multiple biomedical patents. He is a strong advocate for patient-centered medical care, particularly in the field of obstetrics.

www.ingramcontent.com/pod-product-compliance
Lightning Source LLC
Chambersburg PA
CBHW060141130626
46556CB00006B/2444